SURGERY - PROCEDURES, COMPLICATIONS, AND RESULTS

DIAGNOSIS AND TREATMENT PLANNING IN ORTHOGNATHIC SURGERY

SURGERY - PROCEDURES, COMPLICATIONS, AND RESULTS

Additional books in this series can be found on Nova's website under the Series tab.

Additional e-books in this series can be found on Nova's website under the eBooks tab.

SURGERY - PROCEDURES, COMPLICATIONS, AND RESULTS

DIAGNOSIS AND TREATMENT PLANNING IN ORTHOGNATHIC SURGERY

DEVINDER PREET SINGH
AND
SHEFALI ARORA

New York

Library of Congress Cataloging-in-Publication Data

ISBN: 978-1-63482-273-2
Library of Congress Control Number: 2016935300

Published by Nova Science Publishers, Inc. † New York

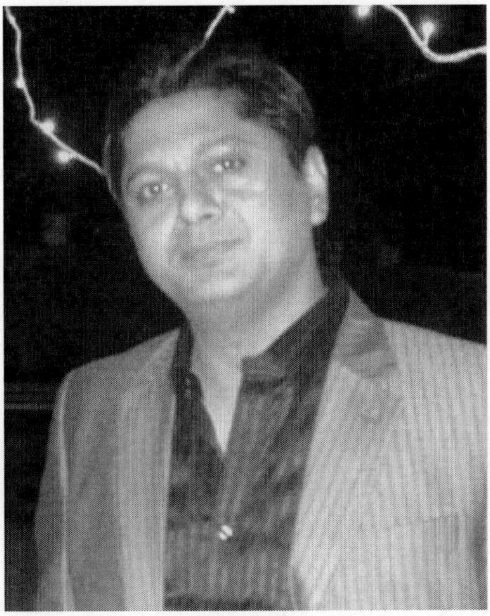

Dedicated to our Dearest Friend & Colleague,
Dr. Rahul Sharma,
who left us for heavenly abode on 07.12.15.
May his soul rests in peace.

CONTENTS

PREFACE

"The human face should be in perfect harmony and balance along with ideal functioning of the stomatognathic system..." a view idealized by Apollo Belvedere, who created the neoclassical Greek sculpture of head and face. But Nature and its vagarities ensure that all of us are not blessed with perfect faces. It is for the resolution of these imperfections, that Orthodontic treatment is sought. But for patients whose problems are so severe that neither growth nor camouflage offers an ideal solution, surgical realignment of jaws or repositioning of dentoalveolar segments is the only choice. Surgery is not a substitute for Orthodontics in these patients, instead it must be properly coordinated with Orthodontics and other dental treatment to achieve good overall results.

With recent advances in surgical technology, it is now possible to treat these patients successfully for whom Orthodontic camouflage would have resulted in esthetically unacceptable and often unstable results. This art and science of diagnosis, treatment planning, and execution of treatment of dentofacial deformities by combining Orthodontics and Oral and Maxillofacial Surgery to correct severe musculoskeletal, dento-osseous, and soft tissue deformities of the jaws and associated structures is called as 'Orthognathic Surgery.'

It should be understood that the technique presented are a vehicle by which a principle is demonstrated. The principle can be achieved by these as well as, perhaps, by other means. It is the principle that is important, the principle as defined within the limitation of our present-day understanding.

References are used where it is believed appropriate and within our ability to document sources of information. It has been our intent to give proper credit wherever possible. We believe the reference lists have scientific merit. While there is much that remains to be known about the practice of Orthognathic surgeries, this text represents a continuing quest for the truth, and our interpretation of the present state of the science and art of dentistry.

We are immensely grateful to the Almighty God who showered us with his choicest blessings and enlightened us to carry out this project successfully. We wish to express our sincere gratitude to our parents, whose unforgettable sacrifices and choicest blessings provided us the opportunity to be educated enough to be in a position to write this current literature. We are also indebted to our son (Angadvir) without whose love, encouragement and support this piece of literature would never have been accomplished.

Devinder Preet Singh BDS, MDS (Orthodontics)
Shefali Arora BDS, MDS (Oral Surgery)

Chapter 1

INTRODUCTION

"The human face should be in perfect harmony and balance along with ideal functioning of the stomatognathic system..." a view idealized by Apollo Belvedere, who created the neoclassical Greek sculpture of head and face. But Nature and its vagarities ensure that all of us are not blessed with perfect faces.

It is for the resolution of these imperfections, that Orthodontic treatment is sought. But for patients whose problems are so severe that neither growth nor camouflage offers an ideal solution, surgical realignment of jaws or repositioning of dentoalveolar segments is the only choice. Surgery is not a substitute for Orthodontics in these patients, instead it must be properly coordinated with Orthodontics and other dental treatment to achieve good overall results.

With recent advances in surgical technology, it is now possible to treat these patients successfully for whom Orthodontic camouflage would have resulted in esthetically unacceptable and often unstable results. This art and science of diagnosis, treatment planning, and execution of treatment of dentofacial deformities by combining orthodontics and oral and maxillofacial surgery to correct severe musculoskeletal, dento-osseous, and soft tissue deformities of the jaws and associated structures is called as Orthognathic surgery [1].

Successful orthognathic surgery demands the understanding and cooperation of the oral and maxillofacial surgeon, orthodontist, and general dentist. Each must provide a proper diagnosis and treatment plan, perform necessary treatment and refer for necessary treatment outside his or her respective area of expertise. [1]. In order for patients to receive state-of-art care when correcting their deformities, the orthognathic team must:

1. Recognize the various characteristics of malocclusion and dento-facial deformity.
2. Define the nature of the problem, including the possible etiology.
3. Design a treatment strategy based on the specific needs and desires of the individual [2].

In this modern era, the role of the doctor has shifted from that of the sole decision maker in the planning process to that of a partner with the patient as co-decision-maker. Therefore, the clinician must not overlook the importance of including the patient and parents in the treatment planning process. Ackermann and Proffit [3] have suggested that clinicians are generally more influenced by objective findings (problem list) and patients are more influenced by subjective findings (their perception of their needs and values). This dichotomy makes effective communication an effective tool when one is faced with the decision between orthodontic camouflage and surgical orthodontic correction.

Chapter 2

INDICATIONS FOR ORTHOGNATHIC SURGERY AND DECIDING THE NEED FOR SURGERY

The basic indication for surgical-orthodontic treatment is a skeletal problem of such severity that acceptable correction is not possible with orthodontics alone. Several factors, presenting either collectively or individually may indicate the need for orthognathic surgery. They include impaired mastication, TMJ pain and dysfunction and susceptibility to caries and periodontal disease. However the most important indication for orthognathic surgery is usually the psychosocial effects resulting from the unaesthetic appearance of a dentofacial deformity [1]. Merely correcting the dental malocclusion does not adequately address the problem; the goals of treatment must include good facial esthetics, as well as stability in the ultimate positions of the dentition and jaws. When a jaw discrepancy accompanies a severe malocclusion, there are three broad possibilities for correction:

1. Growth modification,
2. Camouflage (orthodontic positioning of the teeth to compensate for the jaw discrepancy), or
3. Orthognathic surgery in conjunction with orthodontics to reposition the jaws and/or dentoalveolar segments [2].

Proffit and Ackerman [4] introduced the concept of the envelope of discrepancy to graphically illustrate how much change can be produced by various types of treatment (Figure 1). This diagram helps simplify the relationship of the three basic treatment possibilities for skeletal discrepancies. The inner circle, or envelope, represents the limitations of camouflage treatment involving only orthodontics; the middle envelope illustrates the limits of combined orthodontic treatment and growth modification; and the outer envelope shows the limits of surgical correction.

Growth modification, generally referred to as dentofacial orthopedics, is the most desirable approach to a severe skeletal problem when the potential for further growth exists. Although the pattern of growth can be favorably modified for some patients, the capacity for major increments in growth is rather limited. When a moderate skeletal discrepancy exists and there is no potential for further growth (or if more change is required than can be accomplished through growth modification alone), orthodontic camouflage should be considered. The teeth are repositioned to establish normal overjet and overbite in an effort to compensate for the jaw discrepancy. Such treatment cannot be considered successful if it results in a reasonable dental occlusion at the expense of facial esthetics. In addition, there are limits to how far the periodontium will accommodate the displacement of teeth from their normal positions. The final treatment option for a severe skeletal discrepancy is orthognathic surgery. Once growth has ceased, surgery becomes the only means of correcting a severe jaw discrepancy [2].

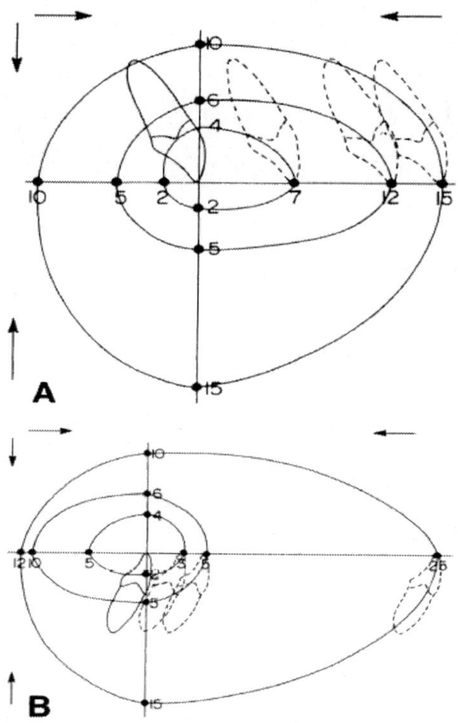

Figure 1. The envelopes of discrepancy, showing the amount of change in the anteroposterior and vertical planes of space that could be expected from orthodontic tooth movement alone (the inner envelope), orthodontic tooth movement combined with growth modification (the middle envelope), and orthognathic surgery (the outer envelope). The possibilities of treatment are not symmetric with regard to the three planes of space.

One answer to the question of "When is a problem too severe for orthodontic treatment only?" is "When the combination of tooth movement and growth modification does not have the potential to bring the patient to normal occlusion" [2]. In a growing child, a malocclusion that cannot be corrected by orthodontics in addition to growth modification is severe enough that it merits consideration of a surgical plan. In the non-growing patient, if the malocclusion is too severe to be treated with camouflage orthodontic tooth movement, then a surgical treatment plan should be implemented to obtain a reasonable result. Merely obtaining an ideal occlusion at the expense of compromised facial esthetics does not constitute a successful treatment outcome.

BORDERLINE CASES-CAMOUFLAGE OR SURGERY?

One of the most difficult decisions that the orthodontist and surgeon face is whether a patient with a borderline skeletal discrepancy can be successfully treated with orthodontics alone [5]. The envelope of discrepancy should be considered a starting point in making this decision. It gives the limitations of orthodontic treatment of whether the occlusion could be corrected, not whether the deformity can be camouflaged. For a patient whose deformity is not within the envelope, the decision must be made in the context of the esthetic impact of two forms of treatment. This is where the patient's input must be sought. Only the patient can decide whether the esthetic difference between surgical correction of the malocclusion would be worth it in terms of the additional risk and cost of surgery. Hence in mild to moderate skeletal problems, patient's opinion plays a decisive role in deciding whether to do camouflage treatment or opt for surgery [5].

Although the patient can and should decide between the orthodontic and surgical possibilities, it remains true that some conditions can be treated better with orthodontics alone than others, simply because the impact on facial esthetics is likely to be better. Profit et al. [6] have provided some guidelines for predicting successful outcome when the choice between surgery and orthodontic correction exists for an adolescent. According to them satisfactory orthodontic outcome is unlikely, and therefore that surgery is likely to be needed for adolescents beyond the growth spurt with a class II malocclusion when (i) there is an overjet greater than 10 mm; (ii) pogonion to nasion perpendicular is greater than 18 mm (iii) the mandibular body length is less than 70 mm (iv) the face height is greater than 125 mm.

In the following table (Table 1) characteristics that can make a difference between satisfactory camouflage treatment and failure are summarized [5].

Table 1. Orthodontic Camouflage of Skeletal Malocclusion

Acceptable results likely
Average or short facial pattern
Mild anteroposterior jaw discrepancy
Crowding < 4-6 mm
Normal soft tissue features (nose, lips chin)
No transverse skeletal problem
Poor results likely
Long vertical facial pattern
Moderate or severe anteroposterior jaw discrepancy
Crowding > 4-6 mm
Exaggerated features
Transverse skeletal component of problem

Chapter 3

PSYCHOSOCIAL CONSIDERATIONS IN ORTHOGNATHIC PATIENTS

THE CONCEPT OF "BODY IMAGE"

Body image can be defined as the individual's composite mental picture of the appearance of his body. Body image has two components: "body sense" and "body concept." The first factor, ***the body sense***, is the actual sensory experience perceived from the body, that is how the person sees himself or herself in the mirror or photograph. The second, and more important, ***the body concept***, is the internal psychological process and sensation that come from within and is an outgrowth of personal emotional experiences; it is the way the patient feels about his or her defects [7]. The emotional experiences a child with a developmental deformity has with his family and society are more important than the handicap of deformity itself in determining body image. If the patient's parents are embarrassed by or ashamed of the deformity, the child will perceive this attitude, and his body image will be made worse than his own sensory input would dictate. On the other hand, if the parents and family provide acceptance, understanding, and a certain amount of protection, the child's body image may remain relatively undamaged. As the child enters the early teens, the influence on body image shifts from parents to peers, but the basic course set by the parents remains unaltered.

PSYCHOLOGICAL PROFILE OF THE PATIENT WITH DENTOFACIAL DEFORMITIES

Face is a major source of one's psychological identity. Individuals are often judged by others on the basis of facial attractiveness; attractive people are perceived to be more successful and intelligent. Such feedback from the society plays an important role in the development of an individual's self concept and self confidence. For people with dentofacial deformities, self esteem may be impaired because of teasing and criticism by others and they are particularly likely to internalize the negative reactions of the others. Children with either severe dentofacial deformities like cleft lip and palate or Down's syndrome, or less severe conditions like extreme overjet, deep bite or severe crowding have lower self concept, are more introvert and neurotic than normal children [8-10]. However after the correction of deformity, others' evaluation improve and the individual's self esteem rises [11, 12].

Motives for Surgery

Majority of patients undergoing orthognathic surgery seek treatment to improve their esthetics or for enhanced appearance as shown by Finlay, Kiyak et al., Flanary, and Jacobson, Heldt [12-16] but desire for functional change is also an important incentive for many surgical-orthodontic patients. The most frequently mentioned reason for seeking surgery was a professional's advice, most often that of an orthodontist while general dentists also served as a major source of advice [2] (Table 2).

Post Surgical Psycho-Emotional Aspects of Orthognathic Surgical Patient

The personality dimensions of neuroticism (the potential for one's emotions to shift suddenly and often erratically) and locus of control (belief that his or her fate is controlled by powerful others) affect the outcomes reported by the patients. The higher the neuroticism score, the more a patient complains about pain, swelling, eating and speech just after the surgery [12]. Overall satisfaction immediately after surgery is however better predicted by patient's expectations of pain and parasthesia than by neuroticism [17]. (Figure 2)

Studies have shown that patients are generally satisfied with their treatment and there is improvement in their self esteem, body image and physiological functions like mastication, speech and breathing [7, 11, 12, 17, 18]. Dissatisfaction is not related to sex, age or procedure rather to their neurotic levels, unreal expectations of post surgical pain, numbness and swelling, weight loss, time lost from work and loss of sensation, inadequate explanation of procedures.

Table 2. Motives for surgery

Parameter	Males	Females
Professional advice		
Orthodontist	83%	76%
General dentist	41%	38%
Other	17%	2%
Desire esthetic change	*41%*	*53%*
Functional problems		
Mastication	41%	29%
Speech	14%	2%
TMJ	3%	16%
Social reasons	41%	53%

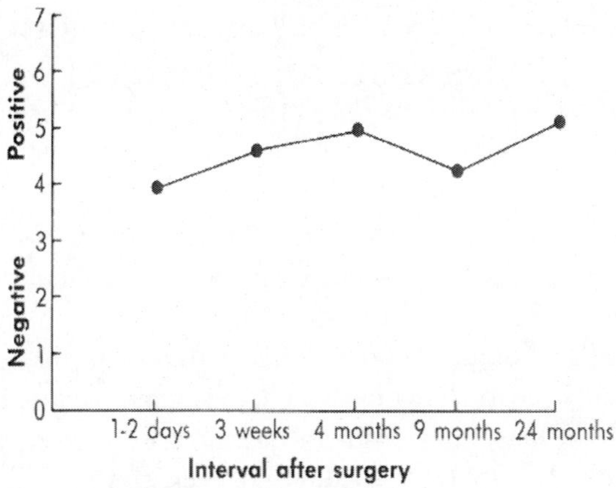

Figure 2. Overall satisfaction with the outcomes is generally high at all postsurgical assessments. A significant improvement from the immediate postoperative stage to 2 years later, with a slight decline at 9 months.

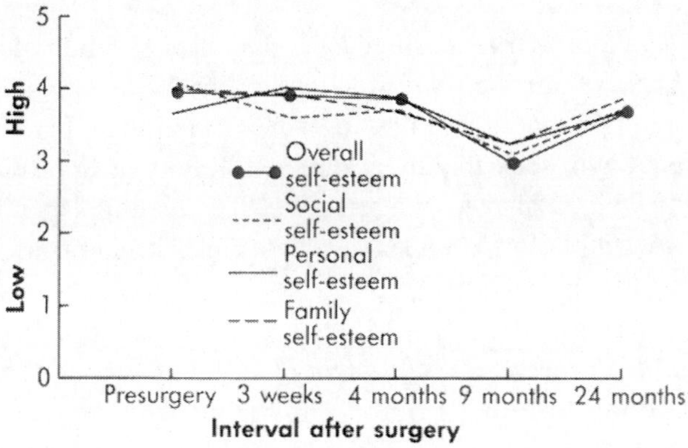

(a)

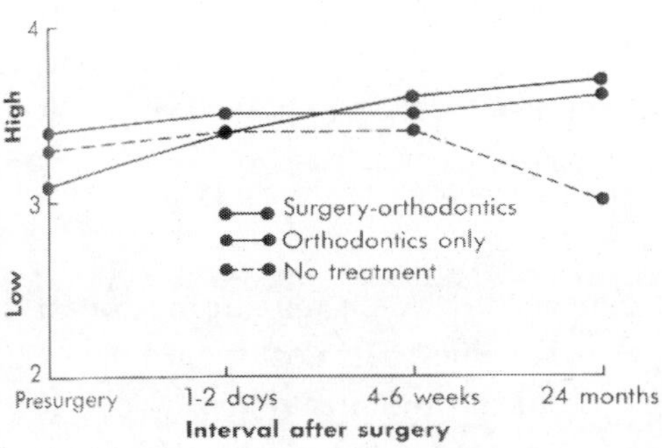

(b)

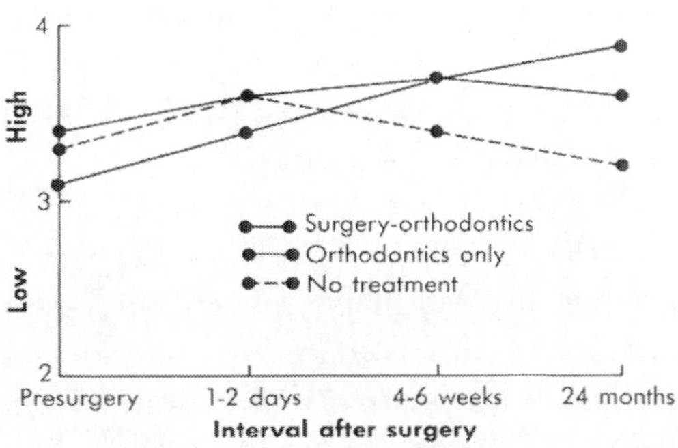

(c)

Figure 3. Overall body image and facial body image scores for surgical orthodontic, orthodontics only and no treatment patients. Surgery patients initially expressed a lower body image and overall image than nonsurgical and no treatment patients. However they showed significant improvement over the next 2 years, so that it was highest after 24 months.

Psychological Evaluation of Candidates for Dentofacial Surgery

Patients who undergo orthognathic surgery may have widely divergent expectations regarding the outcome of the operation. Deformity of the face affects an individual's psyche, particularly the development of body image. Surgical correction of such a deformity influences the patient's personality – usually positively, but sometimes negatively. Postoperative dissatisfaction is usually a result of lack of understanding between the patient and the surgeon. Those individuals who react negatively to surgical alteration generally possess certain personality characteristics which, if recognized before the operation, can indicate that the individual may be a problem patient. The best way to gain the necessary information about a patient's emotions is through a carefully structured interview during which the surgeon clearly defines the patient's psychological status [19].

Interviewing the Patient

The orthodontist and oral surgeon should conduct the psychologic interview used for screening purposes. Lack of relevant information is one of the major causes of error in evaluation, and the importance of knowing the individual patient well cannot be overemphasized. Patients who seek treatment directed largely at improving their appearance are often vain, nervous, apprehensive, or aggressive. It is essential that excellent records of the interview be kept. A simple form can serve both as an outline of information desired and as a record of the data gathered [19].

1. How Does the Patient Perceive His Deformity?

Early in the interview, the doctor must ask the patient why he or she has sought consultation. It is important to hear from the patient exactly what he or she perceives the problem to be.

The severity of the deformity and its relative importance to the patient are also significant in predicting whether or not the patient will be satisfied with the operation. The patient with a large, obvious deformity is generally a more favorable candidate psychologically than the patient with a minor deformity.

2. Has the Patient Had Previous Surgery?

While the deformity is being discussed, the patient may volunteer information about previous surgical procedures performed to correct his deformities. The doctor must note what procedures were performed and, more importantly, the patient's reaction to the surgery. If the patient is seeking reoperation on a deformity that was not corrected to his satisfaction the first time, the doctor should be cautious.

3. How Long Has the Patient been Concerned about the Deformity?

The doctor must determine the duration of the patient's concern with the physical deformity. The longer the patient has been distressed by the defect, the more likely he or she is to accept the results. The aggressive, demanding, and impatient individual who has decided only recently that he dislikes his appearance may be reacting to a stressful situation. A period of concern of *less than eight to ten months* is a negative factor in the evaluation.

4. Is the Deformity Developmental or Acquired?

Patients with developmental deformities generally are satisfied with the results of surgery. Because there was never a concept of "normal" in the patient's body image, he or she generally takes a more passive approach to treatment of the deformity and expects only an improvement in appearance, not a change to normality.

Adverse psychologic responses to surgery following injury frequently occur, even in the well-adjusted patients. Most patients who undergo surgery for correction of acquired defects expect a restoration that conforms to their impression of their body image before injury. The reconstruction desired by the patient is often technically impossible to achieve, even though significant improvements are possible. For these reasons, dissatisfaction with the surgical results may occur. When interviewing a patient about an acquired deformity, the surgeon should be frank about the possibility that surgery will result in a less than perfect appearance.

5. Is the Patient's Motivation Primary or Secondary?

The patient should be able to define clearly the motivation causing him to seek corrective surgery. Motivation is either external, that is, involving the patient's environment, or internal, involving the patient himself.

External motivation is of three principal types. In each, the change the patient seeks is a change in other, not a change in himself. The first is the need or desire to please others. The second type of external motivation is the feeling that change in the physical appearance will make the world less threatening. The third type of external motivation is the desire to remove obstructions to personal or social ambitions that seem to stem from physical flaws.

It is important to ask enough questions to thoroughly explore motivation because a patient whose motivation is primarily external presents an increased risk for treatment in at least two ways: (1) cooperation with treatment and tolerance of treatment procedures both are likely to be poorer than with externally motivated individuals, and (2) there is an increased risk that the patient will be unhappy with the changes produced by treatment. Internal motivation is best; a mixture of external and internal motivation is satisfactory, particularly if the internal component predominates and purely external motivation is a danger signal that should be recognized during the diagnostic evaluation.

7. What Does the Patient Expect from Surgery?

The patient should define what he expects from surgery and should have as clear an idea of the result as the surgeon can present. The doctor must explain clearly what he or she is attempting to achieve, using visual aids such as predication tracings and photographs of patents with similar problems. A patient who has been given a realistic idea of how much improvement in jaw function and physical appearance can be expected will probably react favorably to the outcome. The patient who has vague, nonspecific expectations usually has unrealistic expectations.

CLASSIFYING THE PATIENT

After the interview, the doctor can place the patient in one of three general categories.

Group I – Highly Positive Reactors

Patients can be placed in group I if they have responded positively to all questions. For example, the young man with a moderate prognathism who asserts that he is happily married, who has a steady job, and who simply desires to have his chin made less pronounced so that he will look better is an excellent candidate for corrective surgery.

Group II – Neutral Reactors

Patients who have given mostly positive responses with two or three negative or slightly negative responses belong in group II. An example of this type of patient is the successful 33-years-old female teacher with moderate maxillary protrusion whose relationship with her husband has been strained and who has wanted correction for only a short time. In general, patients who fall into this group require more than the usual amount of attention and counseling during the preoperative phase of treatment to prevent difficulty later.

Group III – Negative Reactors

Patients whose responses to three or four points of inquiry are strongly unfavorable are negative reactors who are unlikely to be satisfied by the results of surgery. The patients considered negative reactors differ from the patients placed in group II because their responses are easily identified as strongly negative. An example of such a patient is an unemployed 35 year old man with slight retrognathia who believes that if his face is fixed, he will able to get a job and to marry. This patient obviously is overly concerned with his appearance, desires correction of the external world, and has only vague ideas of exactly what his deformity is and of what he expects from surgery [19].

Chapter 4

DIAGNOSIS: DECIDING WHERE THE FAULT LIES

Diagnosis for the orthognathic surgical patient begins with the establishment of a data base of information about the patient. Then the process of classification is used to systematically delineate the patient's problems. The resulting problem list is the diagnosis. Three distinct types of information are gathered from an interview, clinical examination, and analysis of diagnostic records to compose the data base. Dentofacial deformities are caused by deviations from normal growth and development and not by disease. An important aspect of diagnosis is differentiating development problems from problems resulting from acute or chronic pathologic processes. The developmental problems are treated by orthodontics and/or orthognathic surgery, the pathologic problems by other means. For this reason, it is necessary to develop two problem lists, one for pathology, and the other for developmental problems. Patients with pathology (e.g., high blood pressure, diabetes, periodontal disease) can have surgical orthodontics treatment, but the disease processes must be brought under control first.

INTERVIEW DATA: THE FIRST COMPONENT OF THE DATA BASE

Information from the interview is of three major types:

1. The patient's chief complaint,
2. Information related to the patient's social-psychologic status; that is, the patient's motivation for and expectations from treatment, and
3. Information related to the patient's physical status: that is, the medical-dental history and related findings [2].

1. The Patient's Chief Complaint

The first goal of the interview is to establish the patient's major reason for seeking treatment, which is the chief complaint as a patient's ultimate satisfaction with treatment outcome often depends upon attention to the chief complaint [20]. Patients who seek surgical-orthodontic treatment – more correctly, those who seek treatment whose developmental problems are severe enough to require surgery, as many in the beginning have no idea that they might need it – fall into two broad groups.

The first group, who typically range in age between the late teens and early forties, are concerned generally about the appearance and function of their face and teeth. These individuals want treatment to overcome a feeling of inferiority or insecurity related to their dental and facial appearance, improve their oral functions, and increase their chances of a more successful life in the future.

The second group, who most often are older, are concerned about a specific health-related problem, usually having to do with potential or actual loss of teeth [2].

2. Social – Psychologic Status

The information sought in the area of social-psychologic status is an extension of the chief complaint. The social-psychologic makeup of the patient is often neglected when correction of dentofacial deformities is considered. Yet this is of importance because, despite objectively favorable treatment results, some patients will express dissatisfaction with their results. This can occur for two basic reasons: (1) failure of the clinician to realistically inform the patient of the probable treatment result (especially esthetic) or (2) unrealistic expectations of the patient regarding the results of treatment. The second reason is most likely to occur in two types of patients: those with acquired deformities and those with external motivations. A deliberate social-psychologic evaluation will help to reasonably assess the motivation of patients. The patient's expectations should be carefully recorded for future reference in planning treatment. Meeting a patient's realistic needs is of primary importance when treatment options are considered.

3. Physical Status: Medical - Dental History and Related Findings

Medical History

The patient population seeking treatment for correction of dentofacial deformities is relatively young and generally without serious coexisting medical conditions. However, this does not diminish the significance of presurgical systemic evaluation and appropriate laboratory studies [21], where patient examination should rule out any cardiopulmonary, endocrine, hematological, neurological, and allergic problems that could potentially complicate the general anesthesia or reconstructive surgery. Following discussion with the patient's physician or other consultation and preparation most patients with coexisting medical conditions who desire correction of facial deformity can undergo orthodontic-surgical correction without life-threatening risks. However, in unusual instances the magnitude of the medical risk may be a contraindication to treatment.

Since individuals with the more severe dentofacial deformities are more likely to have associated abnormalities of head and neck as well as remainder of the body, a comprehensive examination of the head and neck should be carried out. The possibility that the syndrome may be a part of one of the recognized syndromes involving dentofacial complex must be considered, since in many of these syndromes multiple congenital deformities can complicate surgical treatment.

Dental History

All previous crown and bridge, orthodontic, periodontal, and facial pain control therapy needs to be reviewed. Specifically the patient's actual response to treatment and perception of the success or failure of treatment are ascertained. This information is essential in determining the patient's probable biologic and psychological response to the possible correction of his/her dentofacial deformity. But with proper motivation, patients with dentofacial deformities who have badly neglected their oral hygiene take much better care of their mouths and teeth.

Evaluation of Physical Growth Status

An important consideration for most potential surgical-orthodontic patients is whether growth has declined to the very slow levels that are characteristics of adults, or whether significant post adolescent growth is continuing as the growth following surgery is quite likely to cause relapse because the growth pattern that caused the problem in the first place will still be present [2]. For this reason orthognathic surgery should be delayed until growth is essentially completed in patients who have problems of excessive growth, especially mandibular prognathism. For patients with growth deficiencies surgery can be considered earlier but rarely before adolescent growth spurt as continued growth of the normal jaw could again leave the deficient one behind. Example, in case of vertical growth pattern with mandibular deficiency if the mandibular advancement was carried out at an early age, there might be relapse tendency if there is significant forward maxillary growth. So, even in deficiency situations, it is better to wait until after the adolescent growth spurt. Indirect methods of assessing growth status, such as hand wrist films to determine bone age, are not accurate enough to use for planning time of surgery. The best method is serial cephalometric tracings, with surgery delayed until good superimposition documents that adult deceleration of growth has occurred.

Clinical Examination Data: The Second Component of the Data Base

Information from the clinical examination can be divided into three broad areas:

1. Health of the hard and soft tissues,
2. Oral function, including TMJ evaluation, and
3. Facial proportions and esthetics [19].

1. Health of Hard and Soft Tissues

In assessing the general oral health of the patient, the condition of the teeth, their supporting structures and other oral tissues is noted. If the teeth have been poorly cared for or oral hygiene is poor, the first phase of treatment, before making orthodontic-surgical records, is to establish a healthy mouth and improve the home care. The examination of the *dentition* begins by counting the teeth. Any missing or supernumerary teeth should be looked for. Abnormalities of hard tissues such as caries, enamel defects and internal or external resorption, should be noted. Dental infections if present can severely complicate the stabilization phase of surgical treatment and compromise the final result

Examination of the *supporting tissues* should begin with inspection of the buccal and labial mucosa, noting the frenum attachments. Patients with preexisting periodontal disease have an increased risk of disease exacerbation during orthodontic treatment and post surgery, particularly in areas where interdental osteotomies are required [22]. Factors that can adversely affect periodontal health in relation to orthognathic surgery include smoking, excessive alcohol or caffeine, bruxism and clenching, autoimmune diseases, diabetes and malnutrition [23]. In many individuals with dentofacial deformities, the gingiva of the anterior mandibular area is poorly attached and may contribute to development of periodontal problems such as gingival retraction, tooth sensitivity and bone loss.

In such cases, pretreatment periodontal grafts may be considered to prevent creation of severe periodontal problems. Surgical correction of malocclusion is not contraindicated by periodontal disease once an acute problem has been brought under control.

Finally the soft tissues of *the lips, cheeks, tongue, and palate* are examined for pathologic conditions and muscle tone.

2. Evaluation of Oral Function and TMJ

a. *Oral function evaluation:* There are two phases of the occlusal evaluation: function and static. The former is completed by evaluation of the patient, and the latter by analysis of the dental models [24].

Functional Evaluation

The functional evaluation is done basically to determine the compatibility between centric occlusion (CO) and centric relation (CR) and assess tooth wear. Since many Class II and asymmetric individuals have "habitual occlusions, the compatibility between CO and CR must be carefully evaluated. This can often be best done with a leaf gauge. Failure to appreciate meaningful inconsistency in CO and CR may result in significant errors in treatment planning. In addition, tooth attrition is assessed as being absent (0) to severe (5). Severe indicates exposure of the dentin and suggests either severely disturbed masticatory function or significant parafunctional habits.

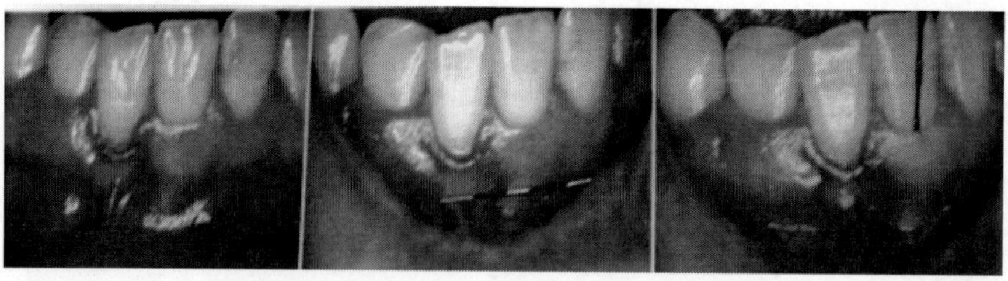

Figure 4. Gingiva of the anterior mandibular area.

Static Evaluation

The static evaluation is performed on anatomically oriented models and is begun by doing an intraarch analysis, followed by interarch analysis and a tooth mass evaluation.

Intraarch relations: The intraarch analysis is done for both the maxillary and mandibular arches. The midline of the arch relative to the skeleton and soft tissues of the face must be noted. Arch form, symmetry, missing teeth, and over erupted teeth are noted. Any cant to the occlusal plane is noted, and the curve of Spee is studied. Finally, the amount of crowding is noted to aid in determining the need for extractions.

Interarch relations: Interarch relationships are those arch relations that exist in all three planes of space. Anteroposteriorly the Angle classification is observed for both molar and canine, and the incisor overjet is examined. The incisor overbite is noted in addition to any vertical dysplasia in the buccal segments. Transverse relationships, including coordination of upper and lower midlines and buccal or lingual cross bites, are evaluated. When a Class II or III malocclusion exists, it is important to note the existing transverse relations when the models are placed into a Class I occlusal relation. This is indicative of the true nature of any traverse abnormality.

b. *Temporomandibular joint evaluation:* It is important diagnostically and prognostically to evaluate the temporomandibular joint. Examination is done in three parts:
   i. Evaluation of mandibular movements,
   ii. Examination of temporomandibular joint symptoms, and
   iii. Examination of temporomandibular joint signs.

If significant abnormalities are disclosed in this evaluation, it is important that the joint(s) be further evaluated and an accurate diagnosis made before instituting definitive orthodontic-surgical treatment of the existing dentofacial deformity [24].

i) Mandibular Movements

Maximal interincisal opening, protrusive, and excursive movements are recorded in this evaluation. The normal interincisal opening is about 50 m; both protrusive and excursive movements are approximately 6mm. if deviations of greater than 2 to 4 mm occur during opening, they are noted and recorded. If opening is reduced or deviations exist, it is important to determine if this is caused by true temporomandibular joint abnormalities or masticatory muscle problems. This can often be simply accomplished by asking the patient to touch the specific area (s) of soreness or tightness that prevent(s) normal execution of these movements. If muscle dysfunction exists, it can generally be eliminated via standard means and the patient is reevaluated after any influences of muscle dysfunction on jaw movement have been eliminated.

ii) Temporomandibular Joint Symptoms

Symptoms refer explicitly to temporomandibular joint pain, specifically localized in the preauricular and external auditory canal areas, as determined by palpation. When true temporomandibular joint pain exists, it is almost always accentuated by movement and by loading of the joint. This latter phenomenon is achieved by having the patient bite hard on a tongue blade sequentially placed in one canine area, the other canine area, and incisally.

When the patient bites in the left canine area, the right joint is loaded; thus biting on the left canines will accentuate pain in the right joint. When the patient bites hard on the incisors, both joints are loaded.

iii) Temporomandibular Joint Signs

A large percentage (30% to 80%) of the total adult population who are asymptomatic have popping or clicking or both on auscultation with a stethoscope. It is important to record if this occurs during the normal functional range of mandibular motion or only on extreme opening. Moreover, it is important to note that most patients who have early popping (before 20 mm of interincisal opening) exhibit an associated premature protrusive movement of the condyle(s) as the pop occurs. In these instances the question is whether the noise is secondary to an underlying muscle dysfunction or caused by a true anatomic internal derangement. The question can often be answered by having the patient undergo 2 to 4 weeks of specified jaw physiotherapy. When this regimen is followed, the majority of patients (75% to 80%) readily eliminate the deviation, popping, and any associated symptoms. These patients have a functional pop and do not generally require other methods of treatment. Those who are not cured by this regimen may have a true anatomic internal derangement and may require surgical or other forms of treatment. Crepitation is very uncommon in asymptomatic joints and may be an early sign of true degenerative joint disease. When crepitation exists it is best to obtain laminograms of the joints to better evaluate them for the presence of early degenerative joint disease.

Predicated on the findings in this examination, when possible or probable organic temporomandibular joint pathology exists, such as significant hypomobility, deviation on opening, locking, and pain localized to the temporomandibular joint(s), further detailed temporomandibular joint studies are indicated [24].

3. Esthetics and Facial Analysis: Deciding Where the Fault Lies

The patient is best evaluated while sitting upright in a straight backed chair with the examiner seated directly opposite at eye level. The patient's head should be oriented so that the clinical Frankfort horizontal plane (a line from tragus of ear to the bony infralorbital rim) is parallel to the floor. The major emphasis is placed on frontal esthetics because that is how individuals most often view themselves and one another. Although the actual details of the esthetic facial evaluation are recorded directly from the patient, facial photographs are essential to document these details. The recommended facial photographs are

1. front face in repose,
2. front face smiling and
3. right and left profile in repose.

Table 3. Frontal and Profile Facial Examination: The 19 Facial Traits Included in the Facial Examination [25]

I. Frontal view
- A. Outline form
- B. Facial level
- C. Midline alignments
- D. Facial one-thirds
- E. Lower one-third evaluation
  - 1. Upper and lower lip lengths
  - 2. Incisor to relaxed upper lip
  - 3. Interlabial gap
  - 4. Closed lip position
  - 5. Smile-lip level

II. Profile view
- A. Profile angle
- B. Nasolabial angle
- C. Maxillary sulcus contour
- D. Mandibular sulcus contour
- E. Orbital rim
- F. Cheekbone contour
- G. Nasal base-lip contour
- H. Nasal projection
- I. Throat length
- J. Subnasale-pogonion line

FRONTAL ANALYSIS

Symmetry, balance, and morphology are the three major elements that are important in the production of good frontal esthetics. Right-left symmetry is studied first. Certainly no face is perfectly symmetrical, yet the absence of any obvious symmetry is necessary for good facial esthetics. General facial balance is determined next and refers to the fact that the upper, middle, and lower facial thirds are nearly equal in vertical height. General facial morphology is next assessed. (Table 3) Once general facial symmetry, balance, and morphology have been assessed, a sequential, detailed study of the facial third is carried out [24].

Frontal View

Natural head posture, centric relation, and relaxed lip posture are used to accurately assess the frontal view.

(i) Outline Form and Symmetry

General outline form and asymmetries are noted. The bigonial width is approximately 30% less than the bizygomatic dimension. Farkas [26] has established normal values for height to width proportion: 1.3:1 for females and 1.35:1 for males. (Figure 5) The important question when assessing these dimensions is: Will orthodontic and/or surgical care necessary for bite correction correct or accentuate existing height and width imbalance? An example of orthodontic correction of height-width imbalance is the use of bite opening mechanics to lengthen the face during bite correction. An example of surgical correction is maxillary impaction to shorten the long face [25].

The most common to least common sites of facial asymmetry are chin, mandibular angles, and cheekbones. The maxilla is rarely involved in skeletal asymmetry. Asymmetries can occur with any growth abnormality but are strongly associated with unilateral condylar hyperplasia.

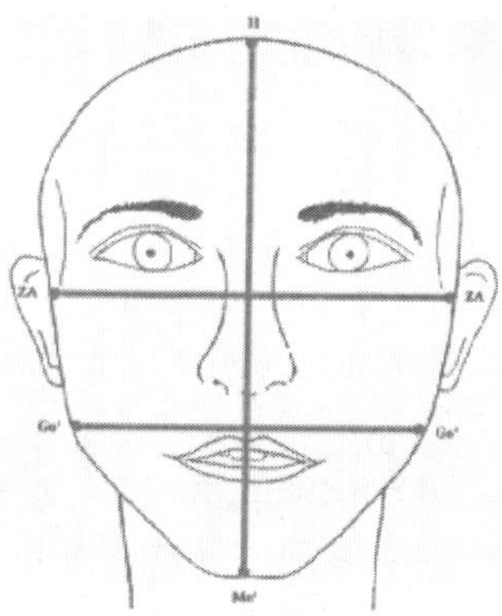

Figure 5. Planes of Facial Symmetry.

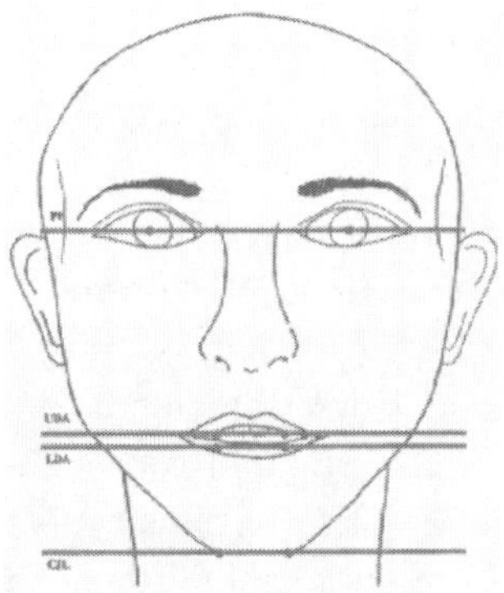

Figure 6. Planes of Facial Level.

(ii) Facial Level

To examine facial levels a reliable horizontal landmark line is necessary. If the pupils are level, they are used as the horizontal reference line and adjacent structures are measured relative to this line. Structures compared with the pupil line are (1) upper canine level, (2) lower canine level, and (3) chin and jaw level. (Figure 6)

Mandibular deviations commonly have upper and lower occlusal cants with chin and jaw line canting associated. Deviations from level should be noted and correction integrated into the overall treatment plan. If the pupils, in natural head posture, are not level to the horizon, a constructed frontal horizontal reference line is used. This line is visualized as follows:

1. Frontal natural head posture.
2. Horizontal line parallel to the horizon through the pupil area.
3. Assess other structures relative to this line

(iii) Midline Alignments

Midlines are assessed with uppermost condyle position and first tooth contact. If occlusal slides alter joint position, no reliable midline assessment can be made. The relative positions of soft tissue landmarks (nasal bridge, nasal tip, filtrum, chin point) and dental midline landmarks (upper incisor midline, lower incisor midline) are noted. (Figure 7)

Filtrum is usually a reliable midline structure and can be used as the basis for midline assessment most often. When the pupils are level in natural head posture, a vertical line through filtrum midpoint is used to assess other hard and soft tissue midline structures.

If the pupils are not level, a vertical line through filtrum midpoint, perpendicular to postural horizontal, is used to assess midline structures. Needed changes are incorporated into the surgical/orthodontic treatment plan to position these structures on the vertical midline of the face.

(iv) Facial One Thirds

The face divides horizontally into thirds from hairline to midbrow, midbrow to subnasale, and subnasale to soft tissue menton. The thirds are within a range of 55 to 65 mm, vertically. The hairline is variable, and the upper third is frequently low range. (Figure 8)

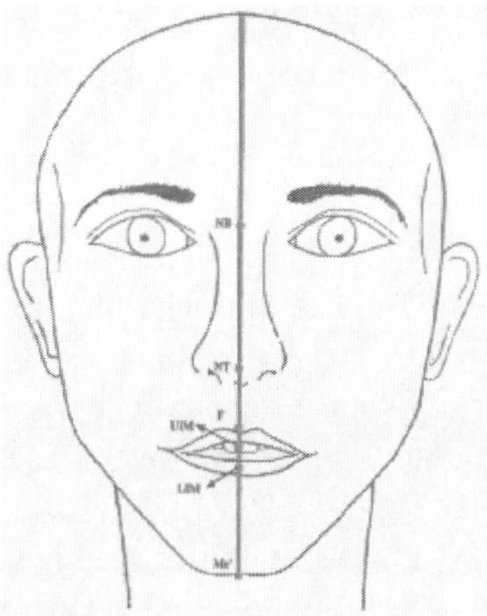

Figure 7. Plane for Midline Assessment.

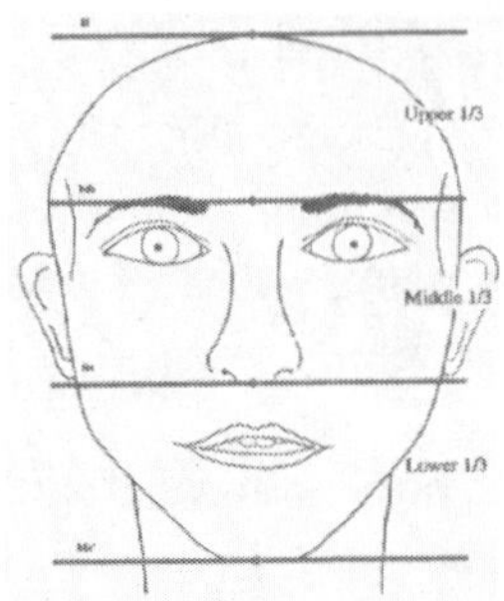

Figure 8. Planes of Horizontal Facial Division.

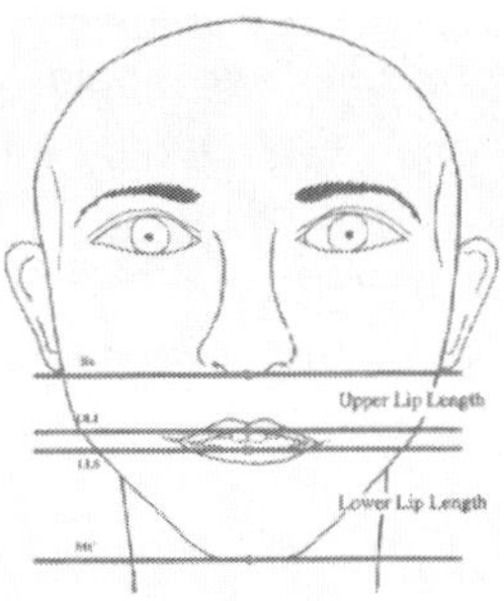

Figure 9. Planes of Lower Facial Division.

Production of correct proportion influences the choice of surgical procedure used to correct the occlusion (i.e., maxillary impaction to correct Class II malocclusion associated with long lower one-third rather than mandibular advancement). The equality of the middle and the lower thirds should not be used as the determining factor in facial height changes. The appearance of the landmarks (incisor exposure, interlabial gap) within the lower third are more important in assessing balance than are the equality of the middle and the lower thirds.

(v) Lower One-Third Evaluation

This area of facial analysis is extremely important in surgical orthodontic diagnosis and treatment planning. (Figure 9)

a. *Upper and lower lip lengths:* The lips are measured independently in a relaxed position. The normal length from subnasale to upper lip inferior is 19 to 22 mm. If the upper lip is anatomically short (18 mm or less), an increased interlabial gap and incisor exposure is seen with a normal lower face height. This should not be confused with vertical maxillary excess (increased interlabial gap, increased upper incisor exposure, increased lower one-third facial height). The lower lip is measured from lower lip superior to soft tissue menton and normally measures in a range of 38 to 44 mm. The normal ratio of upper to lower lip is 1:2.1 Anatomic short lower lip is sometimes associated with Class II malocclusion and is verified by cephalometric measurement of the lower anterior dental height (lower incisor tip to hard tissue menton; women, 40 mm ± 2 mm, and men, 44 mm ± 2 mm). Anatomic long lower lip can be associated with Class III malocclusions. This should be verified with the cephalometric anterior dental height measurement. The closed lip length is misleading and should not be used for treatment planning.

Lip redundancy is seen in cases of vertical maxillary deficiency and mandibular retrusion with deep bite and, rarely, long lip lengths. To accurately assess lip lengths with redundant lips, the patient's bite must be opened until the lips separate. This is best accomplished with a pink base plate wax bite used to open the bite on centric relation (no translation). The face is examined in that posture, and vertical skeletal increases are planned.

b. *Upper tooth to lip relationship:* The distance from upper lip inferior to maxillary incisal edge is measured and normal range is 1 to 5 mm. Women show more within this range. (Figure 10)

Surgical and orthodontic vertical changes are based primarily on this measurement (i.e., postsurgical incisor exposure range of 1 to 5 mm).

Conditions of disharmony are produced by four variables:

1. Increased or decreased anatomic upper lip length (infrequently).
2. Increased or decreased maxillary skeletal length (frequently).
3. Thick upper lips expose less incisor than thin upper lips, all other factors being equal.
4. The angle of view changes the amount of incisor visible to the viewer.

c. *Interlabial gap:* With the lips relaxed, a space of 1 to 5 mm between upper lip inferior and lower lip superior is present Females show a larger gap within the normal range. This measurement is also dependent on lip lengths and vertical dentoskeletal height. (Figure 11)

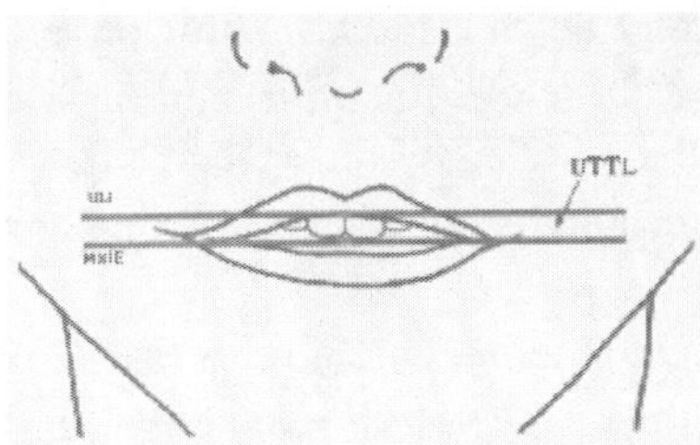

Figure 10. Planes for upper tooth to lip relationship.

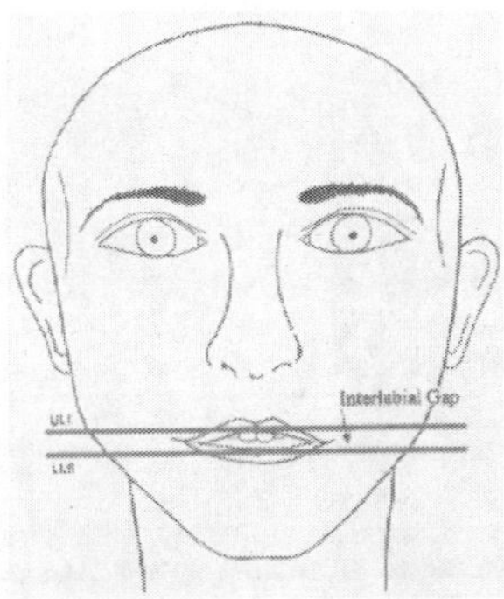

Figure 11. Planes for Interlabial Gap.

Increases in interlabial gap are seen with anatomic short upper lip, vertical maxillary excess and mandibular protrusion with open bite secondary to cusp interferences. Decreased interlabial gap is found with vertical maxillary deficiency, anatomically long upper lip (natural change with aging, especially in males), and mandibular retrusion with deep bite. Abnormalities should be considered when planning skeletal changes. An anatomically short upper lip should be recognized as a soft tissue problem and should not be treated by excessively shortening the maxilla. This can lead to a short, round facial outline.

d. *Closed lip position:* Even though an understanding of relaxed lip position is essential, an understanding of closed lip position adds support to diagnostic patterns. The closed lip position also reveals disharmony between skeletal and soft tissue lengths. (Figure 11)

   Increased mentalis contraction (mentalis strain), lip strain, and alar base narrowing are observed in vertical skeletal excess, anatomic short upper lip and some cases of mandibular protrusion with open bite.

   Lip redundancy is seen with vertical maxillary deficiency and mandibular retrusion with deep bite. With balanced lip and skeletal lengths, the lips should ideally close from a relaxed, separated position without lip, mentalis, or alar base strain.

e. *Smile position lip level:* When examining the smile posture, different lip elevations are observed in normal and abnormal skeletal patterns. Ideal exposure with smile is three-quarters of the crown height to 2 mm of gingiva, females more than males. Variability in gingival exposure is related to (1) lip length, (2) vertical maxillary length, (3) maxillary anatomic crown length, and (4) magnitude of lip elevation with smile.

Excess gingival exposure may be caused by a short upper lip, vertical maxillary excess, short clinical crown, and/or large lip elevation with smiling. Because of etiologic variability, surgical shortening of the maxilla is indicated only when excess gingival exposure is found in combination with increased interlabial gap, increased tooth exposure, increased lower face height, and/or mentalis strain.

Deficient exposure etiologic factors include a long upper lip, vertical maxillary deficiency, and/or minimal smile lip elevation. Decreased incisor exposure is treated with maxillary lengthening when found in combination with decreased interlabial gap-lip redundancy, short lower one-third face height, and normal upper lip length.

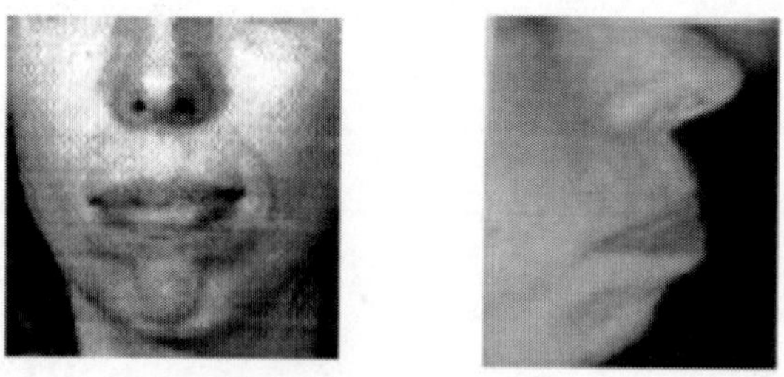

Figure 11. Closed Lip Position with increased mentalis strain.

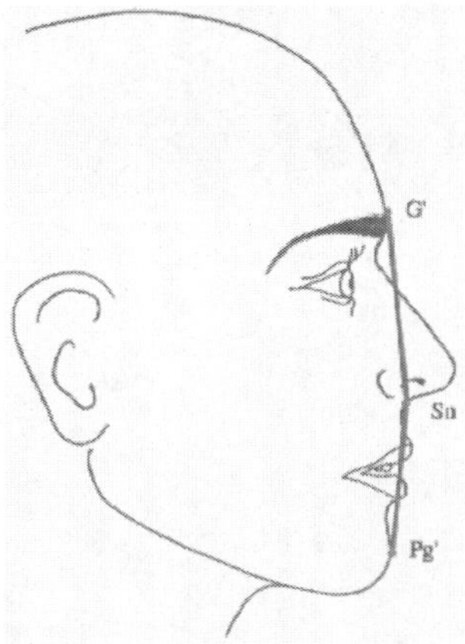

Figure 12. Profile Angle.

When impacting or lengthening the maxilla on the basis of reposed incisor exposure, gingival smile exposure should also be considered. A 3 to 4 mm repose incisor exposure may expose unacceptable amounts of gingiva when smiling because of short maxillary incisor crowns. This situation is properly treated by placing normal length crowns (veneers) on the maxillary incisors and treatment planning from the repose and smile perspective. The "gingival smile" is never treated to ideal at the expense of underexposing the incisors in the relaxed lip position [25].

PROFILE ANALYSIS

Natural head posture, centric relation, and relaxed lips are used to accurately assess profile [25]

(i) Profile Angle

This angle is formed by connecting soft tissue glabella, subnasale, and soft tissue pogonion. (Figure 12) General harmony of the forehead, midface, and lower face is appraised with this angle. Maxillary and mandibular basal bone anteroposterior discrepancies are easily visualized. Class I occlusion presents a total facial angle range of 165° to 175°. Class II angles are less than 165°, and Class III are greater than 175°.

Surgical procedures should generally address the cosmetic imbalance established with this angle. The profile angle is the most important key to the need for anteroposterior surgical correction. When values are less than 165° or greater than 175°, skeletal malocclusions needing surgery are probably the cause and soft tissue thickness differences are not capable of causing these extreme angle changes.

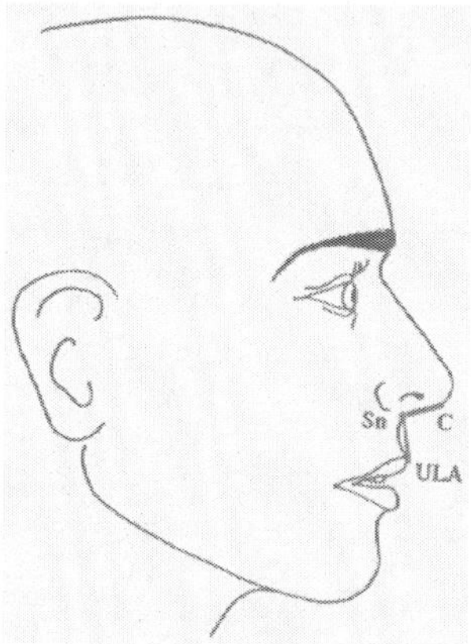

Figure 13. Nasiolabial Angle.

(ii) Nasolabial Angle

This angle is formed by the intersection of the upper lip anterior and columella at subnasale. (Figure 13)

This angle can change noticeably with orthodontic and surgical procedures that alter the anteroposterior position or inclination of the maxillary anterior teeth [27-28]. All procedures should place this angle in the cosmetically desirable range of 85° to 105°. Female patients will usually be more obtuse within this range. Factors to be considered in treatment planning to correctly achieve this angle are as follows:

1. Existing angle.
2. Tilting versus bodily movement of maxillary teeth (orthodontic and surgical) and predicted effect on the existing lip position.
3. Estimation of lip tension present. Tense lips may move more posteriorly with tooth and basal bone movement and less anteriorly. Flaccid lips may move less with posterior tooth and basal bone movement and more with anterior [29, 30].
4. Anteroposterior lip thickness. Thin lips (6 to 10 mm) may move more with tooth retraction movement than thick lips (12 to 20 mm).
5. The magnitude of the mandibular retrusion (overjet). The larger the overjet distance, the more retraction of the maxillary incisors will be necessary, thus opening the nasolabial angle [27-28].

If the nasolabial angle is open (approximately 105°), retraction of anterior teeth orthodontically and surgically should be avoided in treatment planning. Likewise, a long nose will become adversely prominent with lip retraction. Surgical movement of the maxilla also affects the nasolabial angle. As a general rule, the maxilla should not be moved posteriorly in treating dentofacial deformities, especially in combination with superior repositioning. This creates nasal elongation, alar base depression, and opening of the nasolabial angle, all of which create facial premature aging.

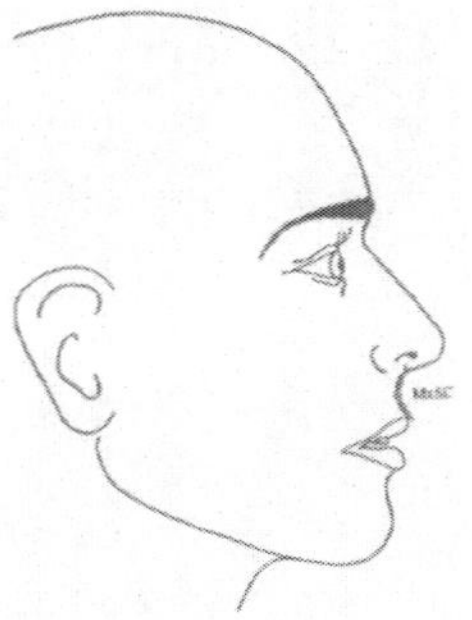

Figure 14. Maxillary Sulcus.

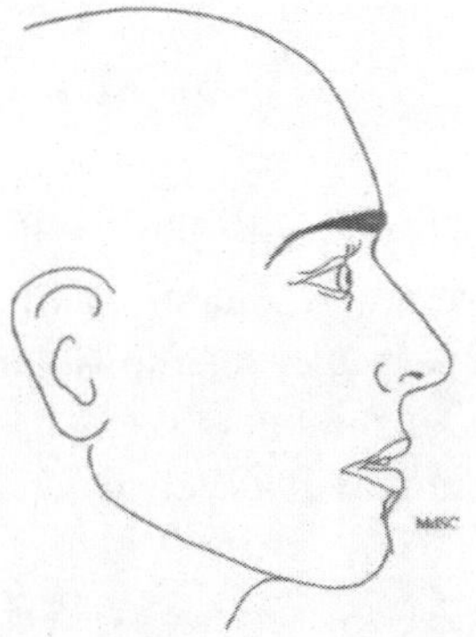

Figure 15. Mandibular Sulcus.

(iii) Maxillary Sulcus Contour

Normally this sulcus is gently curved [31] and gives information regarding upper lip tension. With lip tension, the sulcus contour flattens while flaccid lips form an accentuated curve with the vermilion lip area showing an accentuation of curve. (Figure 14)

The maxilla should not be retracted significantly when a deeply curved, thick lip is present since this produces poor lip support and cosmetics. If possible, the maxilla should be moved forward into a thick, curved lip to improve lip support.

(iv) Mandibular Sulcus Contour

This contour is a gentle curve and can indicate lip tension. When deeply curved, the lower lip is flaccid in character (Class II, vertical maxillary deficiency). (Figure 15) The deep curve is usually secondary to maxillary incisor impingement in the case of deep bite Class II and vertical maxillary deficiency.

When flattened, the lower lip demonstrates tension of tissues (Class III). Surgical procedures that correct the basal bone generally will improve the mandibular sulcus angle.

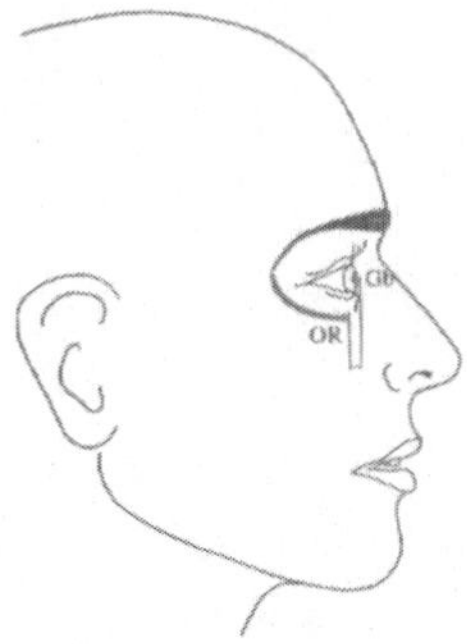

Figure 16. Orbital Rim.

(v) Orbital Rim

The orbital rim is an anteroposterior indicator of maxillary position. Deficient orbital rims may correlate positionally with a retruded maxillary position because the osseous structures are often deficient as groups, rather than in isolation. (Figure 16)

The surgical maxillary versus mandibular decision is influenced by the orbital rim position. Deficient orbital rims dictate maxillary advancement, all other factors being equal.

(vi) Cheekbone Contour

Cheekbone assessment requires frontal and profile examination simultaneously. Cheekbone contour (CC) correlates with maxillary anteroposterior position, frequently the cheekbone contour is deficient in combination with maxillary retrusion. Deficient cheekbones may correlate positionally with a retruded maxillary position. Cheekbone contour is used as one of the main indicators of maxillary retrusion. This area should have an apex at the cheekbone point (CP) and not appear flat. The CP is located 20 to 25 mm inferior and 5 to 10 mm anterior to the outer canthus (OC) of the eye when viewed in profile. When viewed frontally the CP is 20 to 25 mm inferior and 5 to 10 mm lateral to the OC.

(vii) Nasal Base-Lip Contour

The nasal base-lip contour (Nb-LC) line requires frontal and profile examination simultaneously. The line is the continuation of the cheekbone contour line. This area is an indicator of maxillary and mandibular skeletal anteroposterior position. Normal position is indicated by the maxilla point (MxP) directly behind the alar base. The MxP is the most anterior point on the continuum of the cheekbone- nasal-lip contour and is an indication of maxillary anteroposterior position.

Maxillary retrusion is indicated by a straight or concave contour at MxP. When this anatomic area is concave or flat, maxillary advancement is necessary. (Figure 17; Table 7)

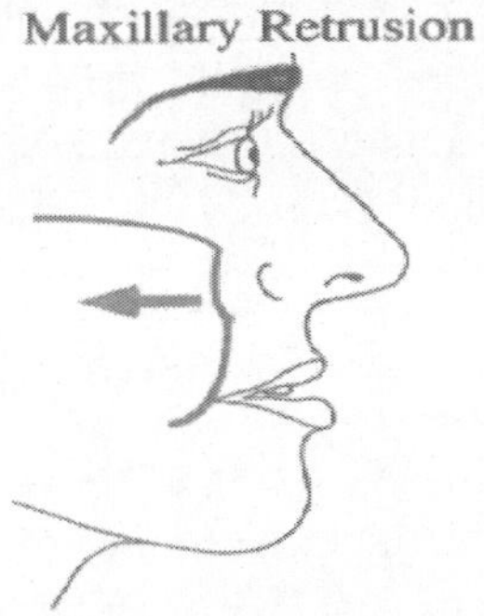

Figure 17. Maxillary Retrusion.

Mandibular protrusion interrupts the nasal base-lip line in the length of the upper lip. When the line is interrupted within the height of the upper lip a mandibular setback may be indicated. (Figure 18; Table 6)

(viii) Nasal Projection

The nasal projection (NP) measured horizontally from subnasale to nasal tip is normally 16 to 20 mm. (Figure 19)

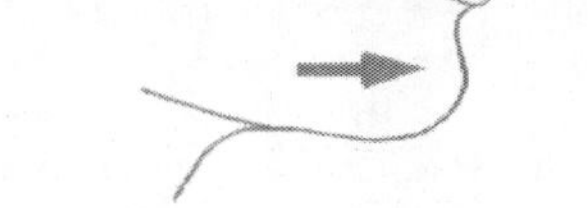

Figure 18. Mandibular Retrusion.

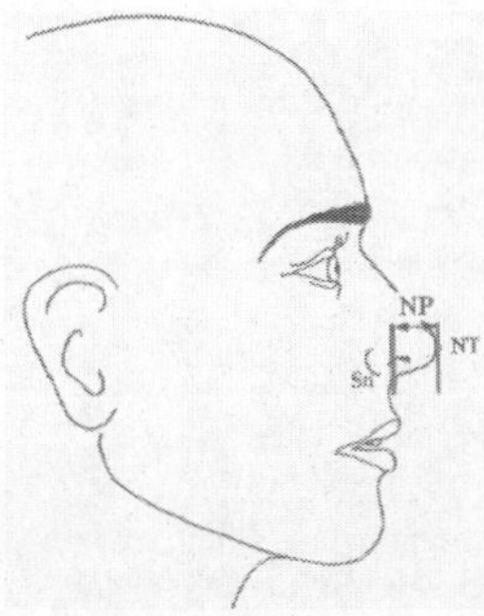

Figure 19. Nasal Projection.

Nasal projection is an indicator of maxillary anteroposterior position. This length becomes particularly important when contemplating anterior movement of the maxilla. Decreased nasal projection contraindicates maxillary advancement. With a Class III malocclusion, short nose, and all other factors equal, mandibular setback is indicated.

(ix) Throat Length and Contour

The distance from the neck-throat junction to the soft tissue menton should be noted. No millimeter measurement is necessary, but a planned mandibular setback will change this length. The predicted esthetic result should produce a normal appearing length without sagging. (Figure 20)

(x) Subnasale-Pogonion Line (Sn-Pg')

The relationship of the lips to the Sn-Pg' line is an important aid in orthodontic soft tissue analysis and treatment. Burstone [32] reported that the upper lip is in front of the Sn-Pg' line by 3.5 mm ± 1.4 mm, and the lower lip is in front of the line by 2.2 mm ± 1.6 mm. (Figure 21)

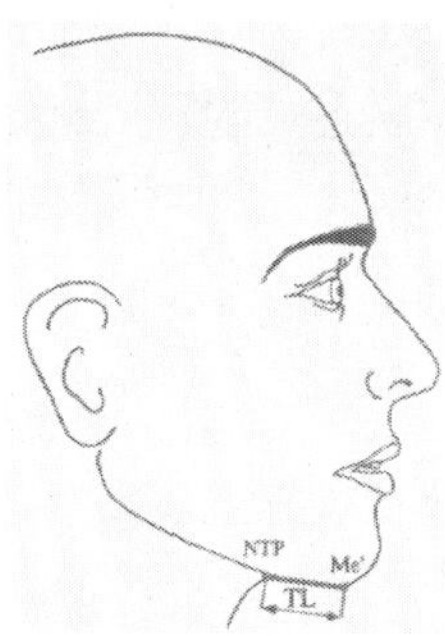

Figure 20. A patient with a short, sagging throat length is not a good candidate for mandibular setback. Often a mandibular setback is necessary with chin augmentation to balance lips with chin and maintain throat length.

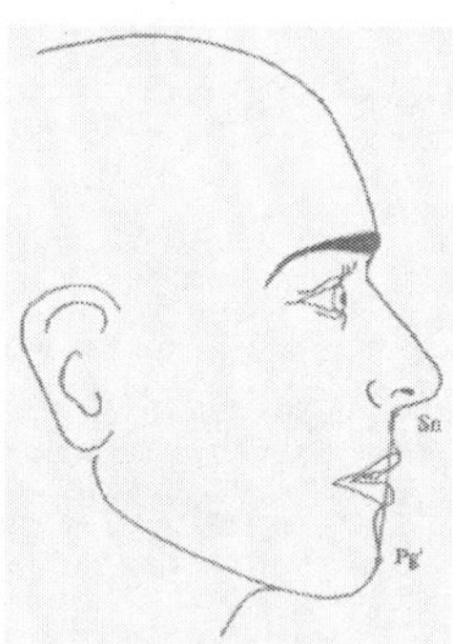

Figure 21. Sn-Pg’.

Tooth movement changes the relationship of the lips to the Sn-Pg' line and therefore the esthetic result. All tooth movements should be assessed in regard to the anticipated lip change to the Sn-Pg' line. Extractions should be avoided when they move the teeth and create retraction of the lips (dished-in) behind this line. On the other hand, if unravelling the crowding with extractions allows for lip balance to the Sn-Pg' line, the extractions are esthetically acceptable.

Table 4. Vertical Maxillary Excess: Common Facial Characteristics [25]

Vertical maxillary excess
Increased lower one-third
Increased interlabial gap
Increased incisor exposure
Increased gingival smile
Mentalis strain
Decreased total profile angle'
Accentuated mandibular sulcus contour
Decreased throat length
Normal nasal projection
Normal nasolabial angle

Table 5. Vertical Maxillary Deficiency: Common Facial Characteristics [25]

Vertical maxillary deficiency
Decreased lower one-third
Decreased interlabial gap
Decreased incisor exposure
Decreased incisor exposure with smile
Lip redundancy
Straight to Class III profile angle
Accentuated mandibular sulcus contour
Normal nasal projection
Normal to decreased nasolabial angle
Increased throat length
Normal cheekbones, alar base

Table 6. Mandibular Retrusion: Common Facial Characteristics [25]

Mandibular retrusion
Decreased or normal lower one-third
Decreased or normal interlabial gap
Normal incisor exposure
Normal smile
Normal-to-lip redundancy
Decreased profile angle
Accentuated mandibular sulcus contour
Decreased throat length
Normal nasolabial angle
Normal nasal projection

Table 7. Maxillary Retrusion: Common Facial Characteristics [25]

Maxillary retrusion
Normal lower one-third
Normal interlabial gap
Normal incisor exposure
Normal smile
No mentalis strain
Straight to Class III profile angle
Normal mandibular sulcus contour
Increased nasal projection
Nasal base deficiency
Cheekbone / orbital rim deficiency
Normal to increased nasolabial angle
Normal throat length

Analysis of Diagnostic Records: Third Component of Data Base

Once the general nature of a patient's dentofacial problems has been discovered by clinical examination, careful study of diagnostic records is necessary to amplify and confirm the clinical findings. Minimum records consist of facial and intraoral photographs, cephalometric and dental radiographs, dental casts, and notes from the clinical examination [2].

Analysis of Photographs

For ideal photographic representation of face, a minimum of 5 photographs are recommended that should be taken with clinical Frankfort horizontal plane of the patient parallel to floor [33]

1. Lateral photographs with the teeth in maximum intercuspal position and the lips closed,
2. Frontal photographs with the teeth in maximum intercuspal position and the lips closed,
3. Lateral photographs with the mandible in rest position and the lips in repose,
4. Frontal photographs with the mandible in rest position and the lips in repose, and
5. A three quarter smiling view.

The smiling view is the most revealing of what the patient actually looks like to other people, and it will disclose the relationship of the lips to the teeth during smiling, which is important for achieving an esthetically pleasing facial configuration. These photographs are intended to capture the aspects of facial appearance already reviewed during the clinical examination of the patient. A photographic examination of facial relationship should confirm the clinical findings. Facial photographs can be used to assess soft tissue chin prominence.

Analysis of Dental Casts

Dental model analysis supplemented by the panoramic radiograph and information from the clinical examination is important in establishing proper diagnosis and treatment goals, particularly in relation to orthodontics. There are eight basic dental model evaluations that should be made [1].

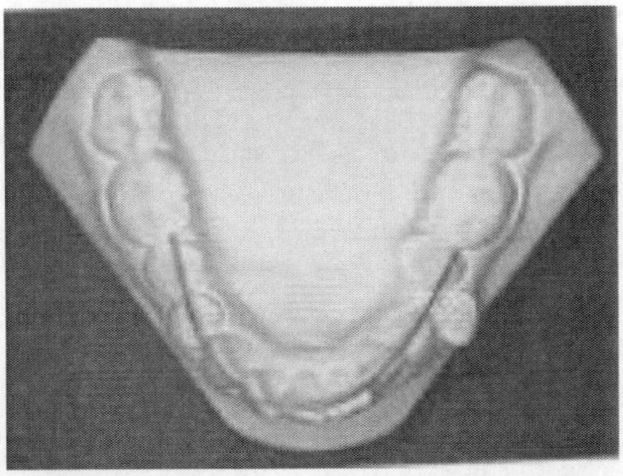

Figure 22. Arch Length Measurement.

1. *Arch length* measurements should correlate the widths of the teeth relative to the amount of alveolar bone available. Evaluation of arch length and cumulative dental widths identify the presence or absence of crowding or spacing. This evaluation helps determine whether teeth need to be extracted, spaces need to be created or spaces need to be closed. (Figure 22)
2. *Tooth size analysis* relates the relationship of the mesiodistal width of the upper teeth to that of the lower teeth. (Figure 23) *Bolton's analysis* can be done to correlate the widths of upper and lower teeth in both anterior region and overall arch. The sum of mesiodistal widths of upper anterior six teeth measured at contact level, divide into the combined width of the lower anterior six teeth, yields a value called as intermaxillary Bolton's index. The average index is 77.5. Tooth size discrepancies can occur in premolar and molar region where maxillary and mandibular teeth should be approximately the same mesiodistal width. These tooth size discrepancies should be taken into account when planning presurgical orthodontics.
3. *Tooth position* in the context of orthognathic analysis refers primarily to the angulation of the maxillary and mandibular incisors relative to the basal bone. The tooth position analysis determines whether extractions are necessary, whether spaces need to be created or eliminated and which mechanics are needed to align and level the arches or segments of the arches.
4. *Curve of Spee* has significant influence on whether the curve of spee in the arches will be corrected orthodontically, whether extractions will be necessary or whether surgical intervention is needed to level the occlusal plane. Correcting a reverse curve of occlusion in lower arch by extruding the incisors may not be stable. To correct this, surgical leveling of arches is preferred. (Figure 24)

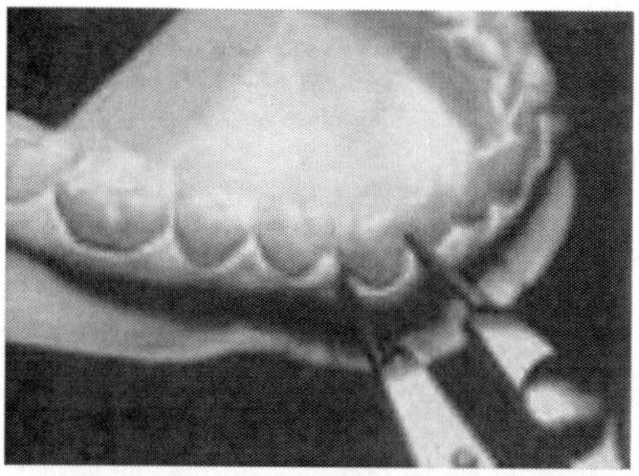

Figure 23. Tooth Size Measurement.

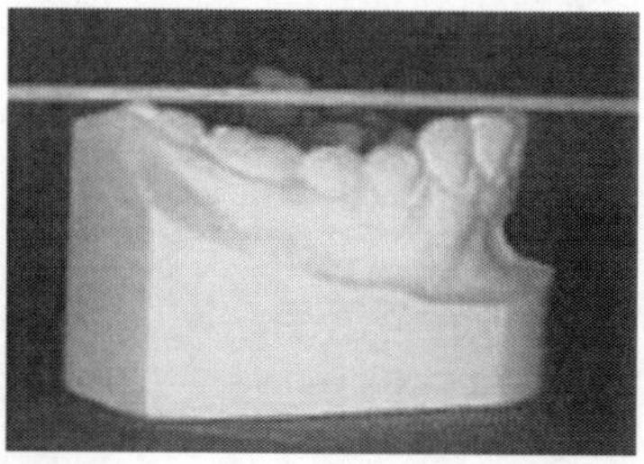

Figure 24. Curve Of Spee Measurement.

5. *Cuspid - molar position* dictates the occlusal functions. It is usually preferable to have Class I cuspid-molar relationship however a class II relationship is also acceptable. A Class III molar relationship is less desirable but may be indicated in some cases.
6. *Tooth arch symmetry* analyses the left to right symmetry within each arch. There may be a significant asymmetry within each arch and correction may require special orthodontic mechanics, unilateral extraction or additional surgical procedures. To determine whether the arch is basically symmetric or asymmetric, one can use a bow divider to measure the distance from the teeth to the midline, or one may superimpose celluloid arch symmetry chart on the occlusal surfaces of the teeth on the cast.
7. *Buccal tooth tipping* evaluates the position of the occlusal surfaces of the maxillary posterior teeth, in a medial-lateral direction. If the occlusal surfaces of the maxillary posterior teeth are tipped bucally, it may be difficult to achieve a proper occlusal relationship. Surgical segmental osteotomy is usually advantageous in such cases.
8. *Missing, broken down or crowned teeth* may influence treatment design. If a tooth is nonrestorable and requires extraction in a potential osteotomy location, the extraction space may need to be closed orthodontically.

Analysis of Radiographs

Conforming Clinical Impressions in Deciding Where Fault Lies

The three most routine radiographs used in the diagnosis of dentofacial deformities are

1. Lateral and PA cephalometric radiographs
2. Panoramic radiograph
3. Periapical radiograph

Panoramic and periapical radiograph can be helpful to determine tooth alignment, root angulation and existing pathoses. Other imaging modalities such as TMJ tomograms, transcranial radiographs, Water's view, MRI and CT scan may be required as determined by individualized patient needs [19].

Analysis of Cephalograms

These are among the most important tools in the diagnosis of jaw deformities. They are used to analyze skeletal, dentoalveolar, soft tissue relationships in the anteroposterior, transverse and vertical directions. However it should be understood that there may be significant differences between the clinical evaluation and the values obtained from the cephalometric analysis. When a significant difference occurs, the clinical evaluation is far more important for treatment planning [34] Analysis can be done either by measuring individual readings or by use of templates.

(i) Measurement Analysis

Following readings are analysed for locating fault in the sagittal and vertical directions [2].

Sagittal

For assessment of *maxilla:* Angle SNA, A perpendicular to N perpendicular distance on the true horizontal, size of maxilla in relation to SN length and placement of its posterior limit with respect to sella.

For assessment of *mandible:* Angle SNB, B perpendicular to N perpendicular distance on the true horizontal, size of corpus with respect to SN length, ratio of ramus to corpus, placement of condyles assessed from the saddle angle and the posterior cranial base length, chin placement with respect to point B and Down's facial angle. (Table 8; Figure 25)

Vertical: Jarabak ratio, mandibular plane angle with respect to SN, FH, PP, maxillary inclination angle, ANS from point N, linear measurements of the vertical development of the anterior dento-alveolar segments. (Figure 26, 27; Table 9 and 10)

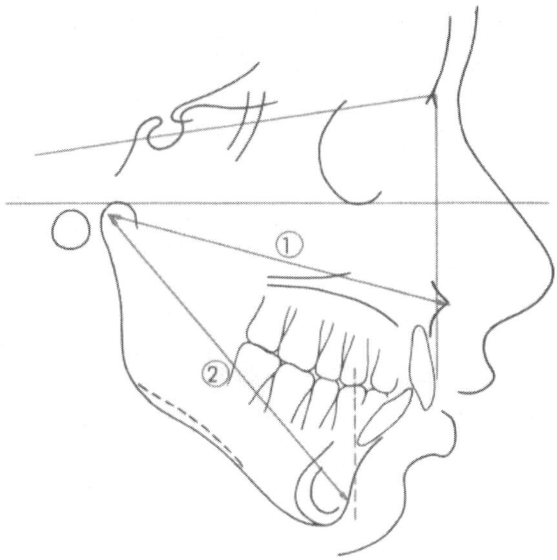

Figure 25. Linear measurements to measure maxillary and mandibular length [2].

Table 8. Cephalometric Linear Measurements for Maxillary and Mandibular Lengths

	Cephalometric linear measurements	Male	Female
1.	Maxillary length (TM – ANS)	114	105
2.	Mandibular length (TM – Pg)	127	119

Table 9. Cephalometric Linear Measurements for Vertical Jaw Proportions

	Cephalometric linear measurements	Male	Female
3.	Total face height (Na – Me)	137	123
4.	Upper face height (Na – ANS)	60	55
5.	Lower face height (ANS – Me)	80	69
6.	Ethmoid point – PNS	55	50
7.	Sella – PNS	56	51
8.	Posterior face height (S- Go)	88	79

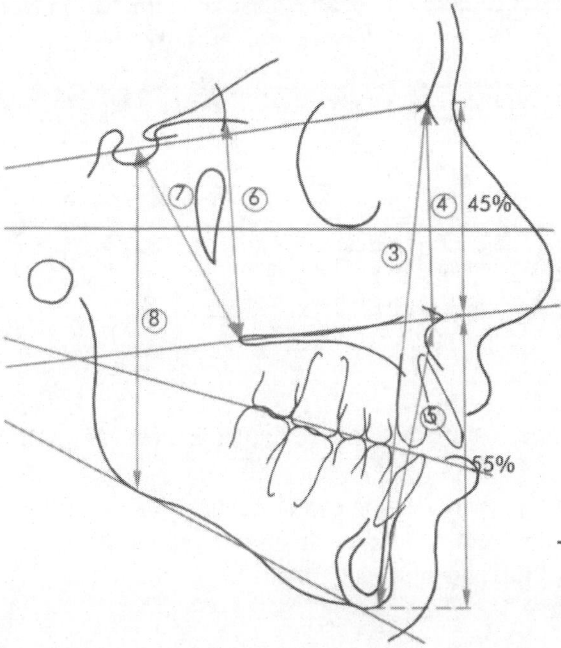

Figure 26. Linear measurements useful in establishing the source of vertical jaw proportions [2].

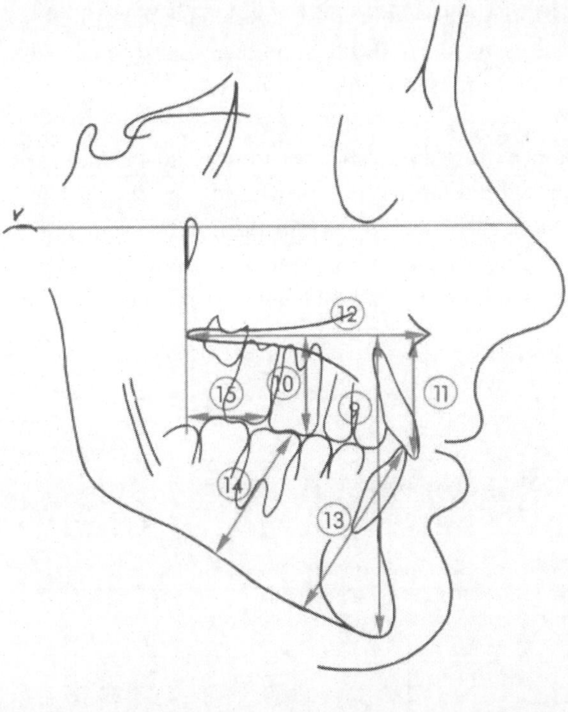

Figure 27. Linear measurements to establish the anteroposterior and vertical position of upper molar and vertical position of incisors and lower molars [2].

Table 10. Cephalometric Linear Measurements for Vertical Position of Incisors and Molars

	Cephalometric linear measurements	Male	Female
9.	Palatal plane – menton	76	67
10.	Palatal plane – upper molar	28	25
11.	Palatal plane – upper incisor	33	30
12.	PNS – ANS	62	57
13.	Mandibular plane – lower incisor	49	42
14.	Mandibular plane – lower molar	38	33
15.	PTM vertical	18	18

(ii) Template Analysis

A template is the visual equivalent of a table of standard values in measurement analysis. As with set of numbers, the template has been prepared to represent the average of a group of reference individuals or perhaps a somewhat arbitrary ideal [2]. The Bolton templates represent the data from a longitudinal growth study and therefore are a series of averages of people from the ages of 3 to 16. (Figure 28, 29, 30)

Template Analysis of Cranial - Jaw Relationships

The first step in using them for diagnosis is to select the template with the S-N distance as that of the patient. If patient's anterior cranial base length is greater than any of the templates, the largest one is used. With the template superimposed on the SN line at N, the antero-posterior and vertical relationships of the maxilla and the mandible can then be observed directly.

A patient who has an extremely severe deformity can be more difficult to evaluate with templates, simply because the template is so different. At first it can look that everything is affected, which makes it hard to decide where the major contributors to the deformity are located. If this is the case, superimposing on cranial base initially and carefully evaluating the maxilla, then superimposing on maxilla while evaluating the mandible can make things less complex [2].

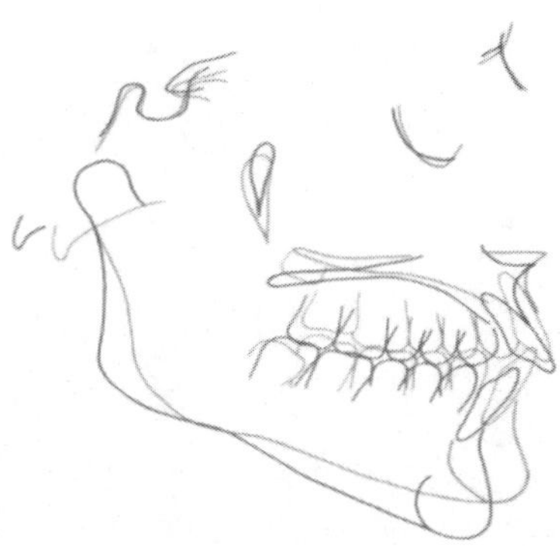

Figure 28. A Bolton template superimposed on the cranial base over the tracing of a 14 year old boy with severe malocclusion.

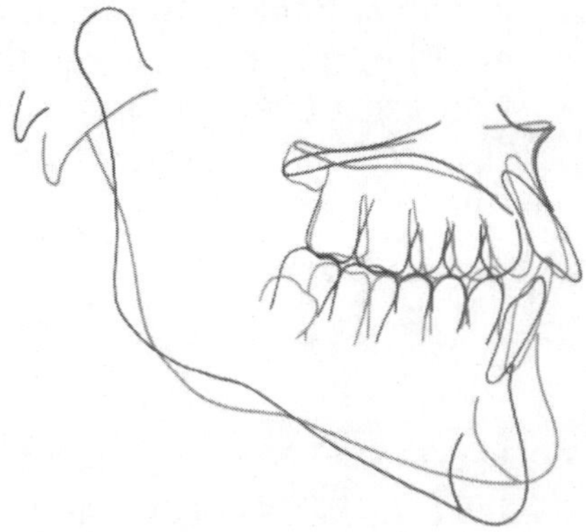

Figure 29. When the Bolton template is superimposed on the maxilla, two things can be observed: the relationship of the mandible to the maxilla and the relationship of the maxillary teeth to the maxilla. a

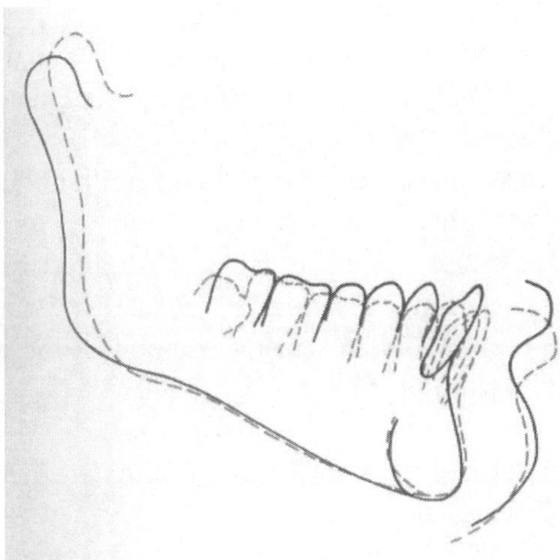

Figure 30. Superimposition of the Bolton template on the mandible shows the vertical and horizontal relationship of the mandibular teeth to the mandible and mandibular morphology.

Template analysis of Dental-Skeletal Relationships: for analysis of the position of the maxillary teeth relative to the maxilla, superimposing the template on the outline of the maxilla provides the necessary information.

For analysis of the mandibular teeth in relation to the mandible, the template is superimposed on the inner surface of the symphysis and along the lower border of the mandible [2].

Quantification of fault from analysis of cephalograms: this step involves the determination of precise magnitude of surgery or in other words by how many millimeters the jaw sizes and/or positions are needed to be altered during surgical procedure. Few quantifications can however be made from clinical examination. For example one of the factors in deciding the amount of maxillary impaction needed is the amount of upper incisor exposure during repose and in smile. Similarly change in alar width, change in shape of nose will be decided clinically.

(iii) Analysis Used for Quantification of Fault Is Burstone and Legans' COGS Analysis i.e., Cephalometrics for Othognathic Surgery [35]

COGS has characteristics which make it particularly adaptable for the evaluation of surgical orthognathic problems. The baseline for comparison of most of the data is a constructed plane called the horizontal plane (HP) which is a surrogate Frankfort plane, constructed by drawing a line 7 degrees from SN line.

Landmarks Used

1. Sella (S): the centre of pituitary fossa.
2. Nasion (N): the most anterior point of the nasofrontal suture in the midsagittal plane.
3. Articulare (Ar): the intersection of basisphenoid and the posterior border of the condyle mandibularis.
4. Pterygomaxillary fissure (PTM): the most posterior point on the anterior contour of the maxillary tuberosity.
5. Subspinale (A): the deepest point in the midsagittal plane between the anterior nasal spine and prosthion, usually around the level of and anterior to the apex of the maxillary central incisors.
6. Pogonion (Pg): the most anterior point in the midsagittal plane of the contour of chin.
7. Supramentale (B): the most deepest point in the midsagittal plane between infradentale and Pg usually anterior to and slightly below the apices of the mandibular incisors.
8. Anterior nasal spine (ANS): the most anterior point of the nasal floor, the tip of the premaxilla in the midsagittal plane.
9. Menton (Me): the lowest point of the contour of the mandibular symphysis.
10. Gnathion (Gn): the midpoint between Pg and Me, located by bisecting the facial line N-Pg and the mandibular plane.
11. Posterior nasal spine (PNS): the most posterior point on the contour of the palate.
12. Mandibular plane (MP): a plane constructed from Me to angle of mandible (Go).
13. Nasal floor (NF): a plane constructed from PNS to ANS.
14. Gonion (Go): located by bisecting the posterior ramal plane and the mandibular plane angle.

(a) Cranial Base Analysis

***Length of cranial base*:** measurement parallel to HP from Ar to N. This measurement should not be considered an absolute value but skeletal baseline to be correlated to other parameters, such as maxillary length to obtain a diagnosis of proportional and mandibular length to obtain a diagnosis of proportional dysplasia. Ar –Ptm is also measured parallel to HP to determine horizontal distance between the posterior aspects of mandible and maxilla. The greater the distance between Ar – Ptm the more the mandible will lie posterior to maxilla, assuming that all other measurements are equal. Therefore one can evaluate causal factor for prognathism or retrognathism. (Figure 31)

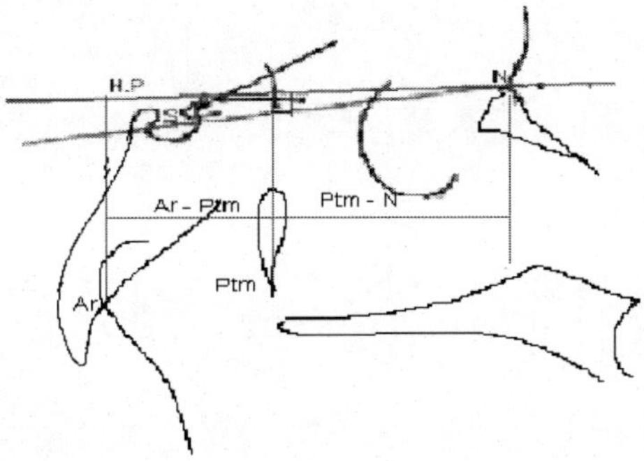

Figure 31. Length Of Cranial Base.

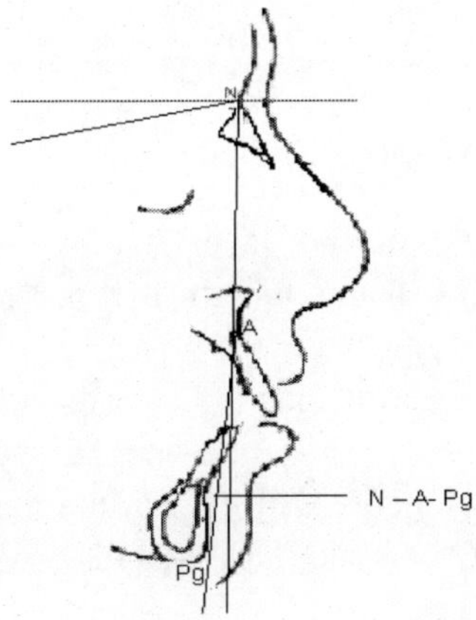

Figure 32. Horizontal Skeletal Profile Measurements.

(b) Horizontal Skeletal Profile

***Angle N-A-Pg*:** this gives an indication of overall facial convexity but not a specific diagnosis of which is at fault – maxilla or mandible.

***N-A*:** a perpendicular line is dropped from HP through N. the horizontal position of A is measured to this line. This measurement describes the apical base of maxilla in relation to N and helps clinician to determine if anterior part of maxilla is protrusive or retrusive.

N-B: horizontal position of B is measured from this perpendicular line. It gives relation of mandibular apical base in relation to N.

N-Pg: it is measured in the same way as N-A and N-B and indicated prominence of chin. Any unusually large or small value must be compared with N-B and B-Pg to determine if discrepancy is in alveolar process, chin or mandibular proper.(Figure 32)

(c) Vertical Skeletal

A vertical skeletal discrepancy may reflect anterior, posterior or complex dysplasia of face. (Figure 33) Therefore vertical skeletal measurements are divided into anterior and posterior components. The anterior component is divided into:

***N-ANS*:** measurement of middle third of face.

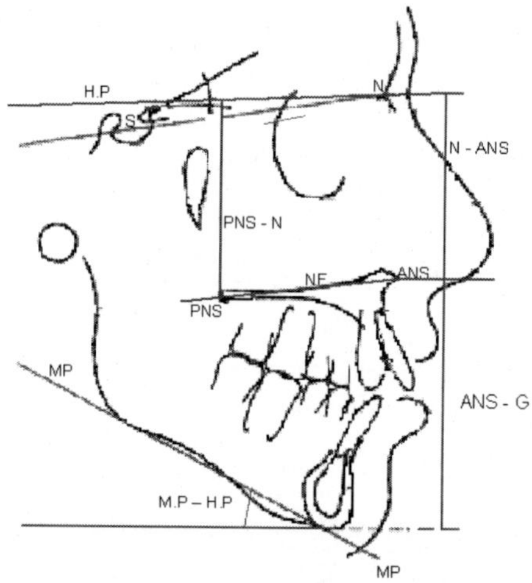

Figure 33. Vertical Skeletal Measurements.

ANS-Gn**:** measurement of lower third of face.

PNS-N**:** posterior facial height that is length of a perpendicular line dropped from HP intersecting the PNS.

MP-HP angle: shows divergence of mandible posteriorly and relates the posterior facil divergence to anterior facial height.

These vertical skeletal measurements will help in the diagnosis of anterior, posterior, or total vertical maxillary hyperplasia or hypoplasia and clockwise or counterclockwise rotation of the maxilla and the mandible.

(d) Vertical Dental Dysplasia

This is also divided into anterior and posterior components.

Upper central incisor to nasal floor: gives anterior maxillary dental height.

Lower central incisor to mandibular plane: gives anterior mandibular dental height.

These two values define how far the incisors have erupted in relation to nasal floor and mandibular plane respectively.

Upper first molar to nasal floor: gives posterior upper dental height. ***Lower first molar to mandibular plane***: gives posterior lower dental height.

These values should be related to ANS-Gn and MP-HP to determine whether the origin of maxillary and mandibular discrepancies is skeletal, dental or a combination of both.

(e) Maxilla and Mandible Analysis

PNS-ANS: gives total maxillary length.

Ar-Go: gives the length of mandibular ramus

Go-Pg: gives total mandibular body length.

Ar-Go-Gn angle: gonion angle that represents the relationship between the ramal plane and MP.

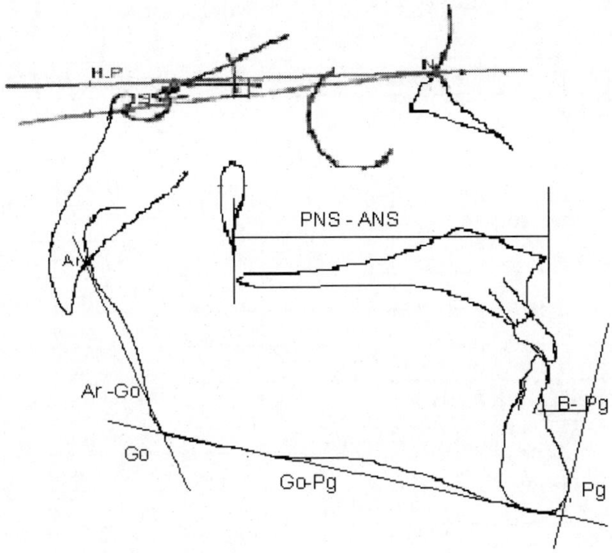

Figure 34. Maxilla and Mandible Analysis.

These measurements are helpful in the diagnosis of variations in ramus height that effect open bite or deep bite problems, increased or decreased mandibular body length, acute to obtuse gonial angles that also contribute to skeletal open or closed bite. (Figure 34)

(f) Dental Analysis

O.P to H.P angle: angle formed between occlusal plane and horizontal plane. Increased OP-HP value may be associated with skeletal open bite, lip incompetence, increased facial angle, retrognathia or increased MP angle. Decreased OP angle value may be associated with a deep bite, decreased facial height, or lip redundancy.

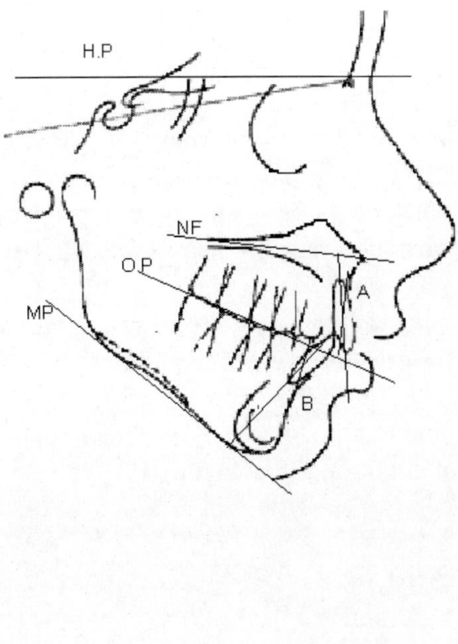

Figure 35. Dental Analysis.

Table 11. Table of Measurements

	Standard (male)	S.D	Standard (F)	S.D
Cranial base				
Ar-Ptm	*37.1mm*	*2.8*	*32.8 mm*	*1.9*
Ptm-N	*52.8mm*	*4.1*	*50.9mm*	*3*
Horizontal(skeletal)				
N-A-Pg angle	*3.9°*	*6.4°*	*2.6°*	*5.1°*
N-A	*0.0mm*	*3.7*	*-2mm*	*3.7*
N-B	*-5.3mm*	*6.7*	*-6.9mm*	*4.3*
N-Pg	*-4.3mm*	*8.5*	*-6.5mm*	*5.1*
Vertical (skeletal, dental)				
N-ANS	*54.7 mm*	*3.2*	*50 mm*	*2.4*
ANS-Gn	*68.6 mm*	*3.8*	*61.3 mm*	*3.3*
PNS-N	*53.9 mm*	*1.7*	*50.6 mm*	*2.2*
MP-HP angle	*23°*	*5. 9°*	*24. 2°*	*5°*
Upper 1- NF	*30.5 mm*	*2.1*	*27.5 mm*	*1.7*
Lower1- MP	*45 mm*	*2.1*	*40.8*	*1.8*
Upper 6- NF	*26.2mm*	*2*	*23mm*	*1.3*
Lower 6 – MP	*35.8mm*	*2.6*	*32.1mm*	*1.9*
Maxilla, Mandible				
PNS-ANS	*57.7mm*	*2.5*	*52.6mm*	*3.5*
Ar-Go	*52mm*	*4.2*	*46.8mm*	*2.5*
Go-Pg	*83.7mm*	*4.6*	*74.3mm*	*5.8*
B-Pg	*8.9mm*	*1.7*	*7.2mm*	*1.9*
Ar-Go-Gn	*119.1°*	*6.5°*	*122°*	*6.9°*
Dental				
OP- HP	*6.2°*	*5.1°*	*7.1°*	*2.5°*
A-B	*-1.1mm*	*2*	*-0.4mm*	*2.5*
Upper 1 – NF angle	*111°*	*4.7°*	*112.5°*	*5. 3°*
Lower 1 – MP angle	*95.9°*	*5.2°*	*95.9°*	*5.7°*

A-B: measured by dropping perpendiculars from A and B respectively on occlusal plane and linear distance measured. This gives the relationship of maxillary and mandibular apical base to the O.P. If A-B distance is large with point B projected posteriorly to point A, mandibular denture base discrepancy that predisposes to skeletal class II malocclusion is present.

Upper incisor to nasal floor (angle): gives angulation of maxillary central incisor to NF.

Lower incisor to mandibular plane: gives angulation of mandibular central incisor to MP.

These angulations determine the procumbency or recumbancy of incisor and are vital in assessing long term stability of dentition [35]. (Figure 35)

Chapter 5

DERIVING A DIAGNOSTIC LIST

Before developing a treatment plan, establish a list of all existing problems evident from clinical, radiographic, study models, and all other indicated evaluations. This problem list should include:

1. Skeletal imbalances
2. Occlusal problems
3. Aesthetic concerns
4. TMJ and/or myofacial pain
5. Missing teeth, crowns, bridges, endodontically treated teeth, dental implants
6. Periodontal problems
7. Other functional disorders [1]

The diagnostic list includes all functional, aesthetic and dental problems as well any other medical factors that may affect treatment outcomes. Then this problem list is placed in priority order. Deciding what is most important for an individual patient should be based on the patient's concerns and the clinician's best judgment. The treatment plan is then formulated from the problem list taking one problem at a time.

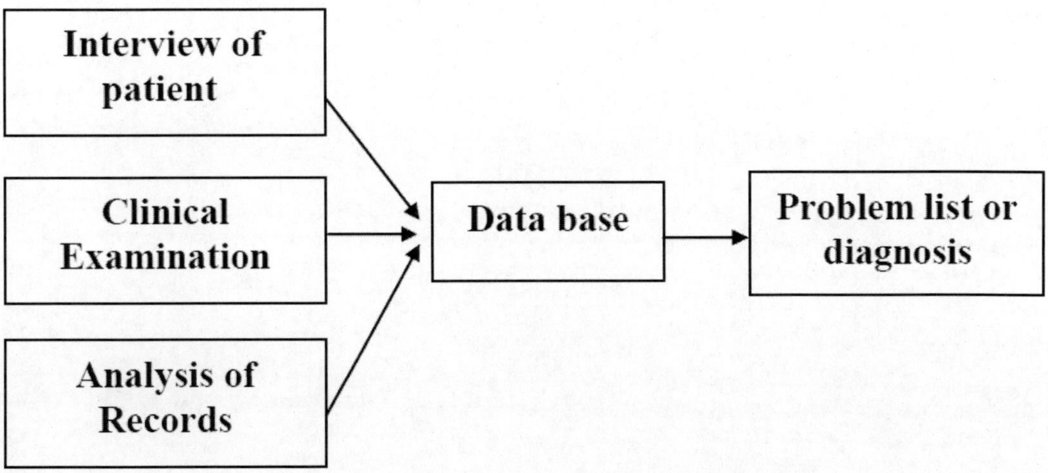

Chapter 6

Surgical Treatment Possibilities

It is not possible to begin planning surgical orthodontic treatment without considering what the possibilities are for treatment [30].

Changes in Width of the Maxilla

Surgically it is possible both to widen and to narrow the maxilla. (Figure 36) Narrowing is technically more difficult because it is necessary to remove bone to bring the two sides closer together, but this movement is entirely feasible. Healing occurs at faster rate when maxilla is widened and graft may be occasionally required. The major constraints on transverse changes are the palatal soft tissues and to a lesser extent the soft tissues laterally and superiorly. Maxilla can be successfully widened on an average of 10mm and 15 mm at the extreme. When planning for maxillary widening, stability of the repositioned segments should be considered and there is a relapse tendency in 2 ways:

i. Two halves tend to move back even if a graft fills the gap and the position of the teeth is maintained.
ii. There is a tendency toward dental relapse after the fixation is removed

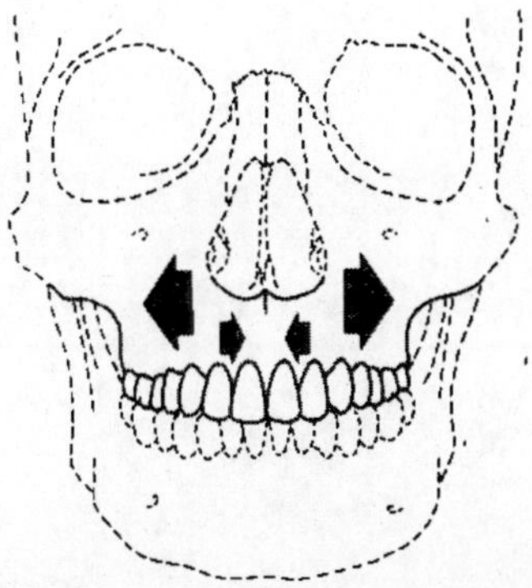

Figure 36. Surgically it is possible to both widen and narrow the maxilla. As the figure suggests widening is more easily accomplished than narrowing.

This combination leads to 40% decrease in intermolar width that was established at surgery [36].

Changes in Width of the Mandible

Changes in width of the mandible are not easy as maxillary width changes (Figure 37). There are two major limitations:

1. Soft tissue envelope.
2. Temporo-mandibular joint.

Antero-Posterior and Vertical Changes in Maxilla

Surgically the entire maxilla can be moved upward and forward with good stability. (Figure 38) The key to success is an osteotomy that frees it from its posterior and superior attachments. When this has been accomplished the maxilla can be moved forward up to 10 mm with good stability.

Forward Movement

This movement has 2 limitations

1. Major limitation to move the maxilla forward is the resistance of the soft tissues anterior to it (upper lip). It is particularly important in a patient with cleft lip and palate who is likely to have maxillary deficiency and good candidate for maxillary advancement.

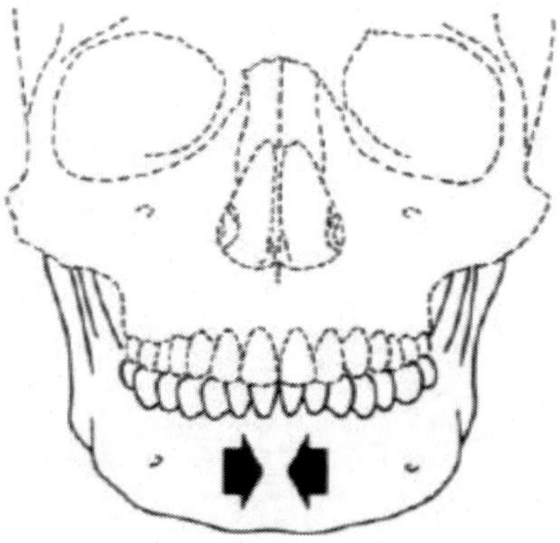

Figure 37. Surgically it is possible to narrow the width of the mandible anteriorly but for all practical purposes it is impossible to widen it as it is extremely difficult to obtain adequate soft tissue coverage of bone graft.

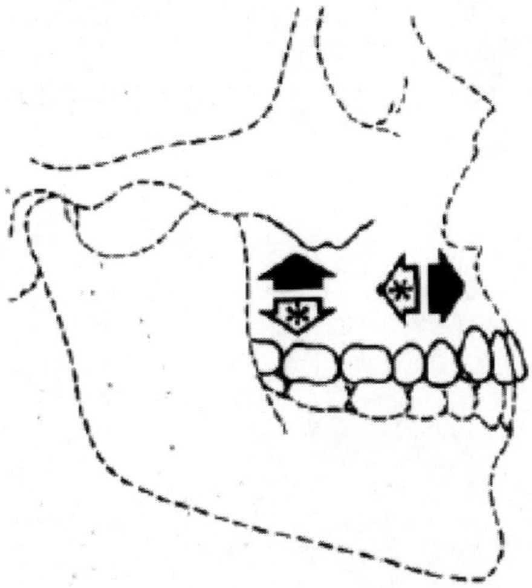

Figure 38. Surgically it is quite feasible to move the entire maxilla upward or forward. It is difficult to move it backward because of the structures behind it and difficult to move it downward because of postsurgical instability.

2. Velopharyngeal closure during speech: Failure to achieve a seal to between soft palate and the posterior pharyngeal wall allows leakage of air through the nose and causes "cleft-palate speech" in normal patients.

Backward Movement

Very limited movement is possible (only 3-5mm) due to bony interferences. Instead the objective is to retract the protruding anterior portion by sectioning the maxilla and removing the bone across the palate. Then the anterior segments can be brought back posteriorly while the posterior segments remain in position.

Upward Movement

When the maxilla is moved up, it does not tend to come back down and is indeed remarkably stable in its superior position [37]. Also the mandible rotates up along with it, and the surgical results are remarkably stable. Neuro-muscular adaptation must occur to change the postural position of the mandible. If it did not occur, there would be no decrease in face height, just an increase in freeway space between the teeth and jaws in its postural position.

Downward Movement

Inter-positional grafts are required to prevent the relapse tendency during this movement. Instability may be due to the stretch of the soft tissues created when the maxilla is moved downward. This would create a gentle and constant force to move the maxilla back [34].

Additional fixation with graft materials is required to stabilize the maxilla and mandible against vertical changes (mechanical stability).

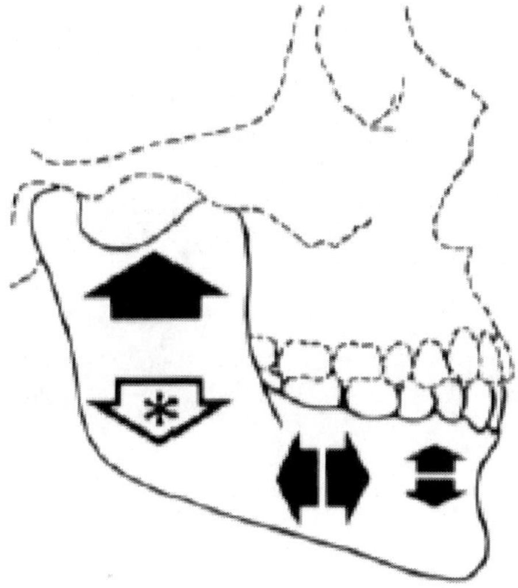

Figure 39. Anterioposterior and vertical changes in the mandible.

Antero-Posterior and Vertical Changes in Mandible

Mandible can be moved forward or backward anteriorly and down or up anteriorly but only upward at gonial region. (Figure 39) Chin can be moved in all three planes of space. Vertical changes also will occur along with horizontal movements and the vertical changes are primary determinants of post surgical stability. When the mandible is moved forward or backward, there are 3 possibilities for vertical reorientation.

1. The mandibular plane increases as the chin moves down and gonial angles moves up.
2. It can remain same
3. It can decrease as the chin moves up and the gonial angles moves down.

This rotational pattern has major effect on post surgical stability [38].

1. Increase in mandibular plane has a greater stability.
2. Changes along the plane are not very stable but acceptable.
3. Decrease in the mandibular plane is unstable and should be avoided.

Soft tissue stretch is also considerable to be one of the causes of instability. So, a better stability can be expected when the mandible is set back than advanced because soft tissue stretching causes relapse in advancement where as relaxation of muscles in setback contributes for stability [2].

Chapter 7

TREATMENT PLANNING

The goal of treatment planning is to develop the plan that will maximize benefit to the patient. As a result of the systematic evaluation of the patient with dentofacial deformity the various problems related to the patient's treatment are clearly identified. If an important diagnostic point has been missed, the treatment plan is likely to be seriously flawed [4].

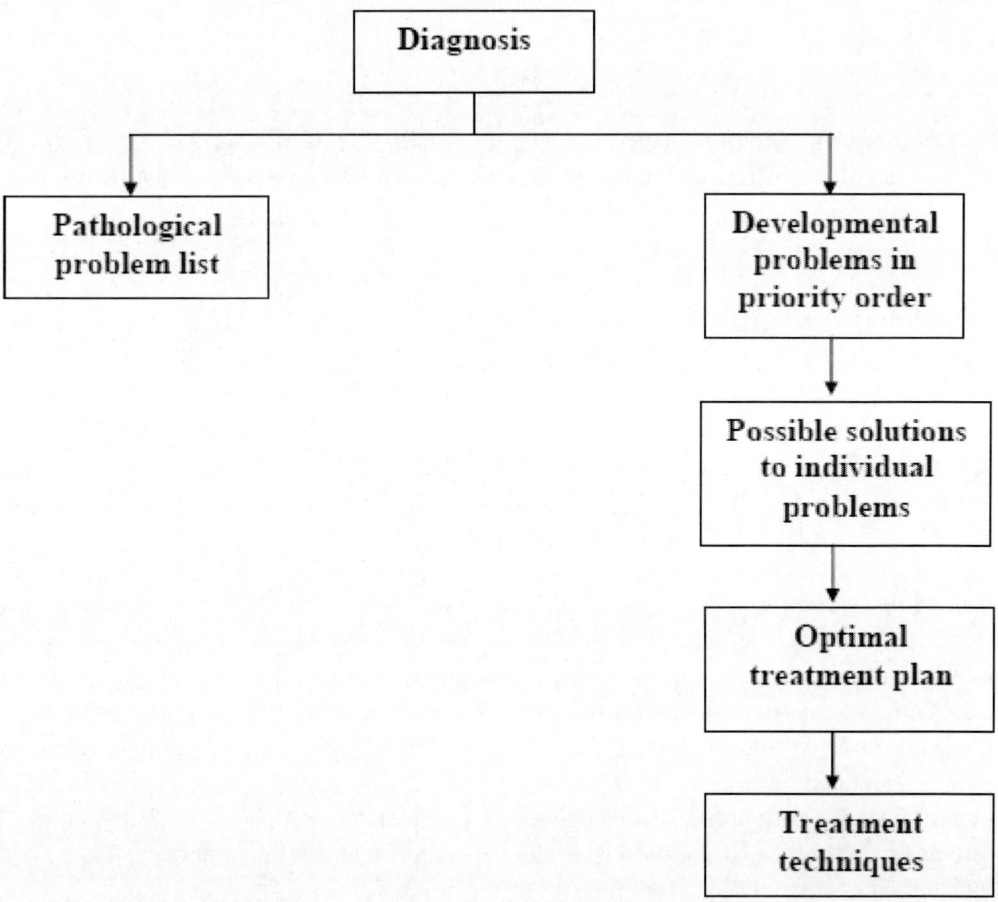

There are three basic questions that must be answered in planning for combined orthodontic-surgical treatment.

1. What surgical procedure(s) is (are) most appropriate for the patient.
2. What specific orthodontic treatment is necessary in conjunction with the proposed surgery?
3. What will be the sequence in combining the orthodontics and surgery [24]?

1. Making the Basic Surgical Decisions

The primary surgical procedure is predicted upon the existing facial esthetics and the patient's desired change(s) in them. Once the esthetic problems are defined, the type of surgical procedure(s) to be performed for a given patient is readily determined. For example, for a patient whose only esthetic problem is recessive chin, the esthetic treatment objective would be to increase the chin prominence. Therefore only two surgical procedures could be considered: advancing the mandible or augmentation genioplasty. Which of these procedures or possibly both would be done is then determined from

1. Evaluation of the occlusion and
2. Cephalometric prediction tracings [24]

Nevertheless, the primary surgical procedure is predicted on the existing facial esthetics alone. Analysis of occlusion and cephalometric prediction tracings are needed to determine the details of the surgery and the need for adjunctive surgical procedures.

Esthetic Treatment Objectives

The basic surgical decision is made as a direct extension of the esthetic facial evaluation and the resulting esthetic treatment objectives and modified by integration of the occlusal findings and cephalometric prediction tracing results. However it is important that despite profile esthetic treatment objectives, front face esthetics are more important and must never be worsened as a result of the surgical procedure [24].

Integration of Occlusion

Decisions based on the present occlusion are important in those patients for whom there is more than one surgical procedure that will accomplish the desired facial esthetic change. In such cases, the choice of a specific procedure will be based on determining which of the possible procedures will produce the best occlusal result. For example, in a patient for whom the esthetic treatment objective is to increase chin prominence, several details must be determined. If such a patient has a satisfactory and stable occlusion, augmentation genioplasty is the treatment of choice. If patient has a class II malocclusion, a mandibular advancement with or without augmentation genioplasty is most optimal. Finally, additional questions regarding the specifics of the indicated surgical procedure(s) require cephalometric prediction tracings.

Integration of prediction tracings

Once the basic surgical decision has been made, prediction tracings are used to determine the effect of the proposed surgery on profile esthetics. Importantly these prediction tracings are *not* done at this time to plan the magnitude of surgical procedure, but to determine:

1. If the surgical procedure will indeed produce the desired facial esthetic changes.
2. If such a procedure is possible within the limitations of good surgical technique.
3. If the orthodontic treatment called for in conjunction with the proposed surgery is feasible

An accurate prediction tracing is a necessary tool for the orthodontist because it allows him to discern the anterior-posterior dental compensations present in a given malocclusion, and plan orthodontic treatment which will effectively eliminate these compensations, thus allowing the surgeon to effect the desired esthetic result One last benefit can be derived from these detailed prediction tracings and this is in the area of consultation. With an accurate tracing, one can, in effect, show patients and their parents the proposed treatment results, at least in profile, which should allow them to better understand and more readily accept the proposed treatment [24].

There are five general methods of visualizing, planning, and predicting surgical orthodontic outcomes [39]:

1. Manual acetate tracing "cut and paste" techniques.
2. Manipulation of patient photographs to illustrate treatment goals.
3. Computerized diagnostic and planning software that produces a soft tissue profile “line drawing”; as a result of manipulation of digitized structures of lateral cephalometric radiographs.
4. Computerized diagnostic and planning software that integrates video images with the patient's lateral cephalogram to aid in planning and predicting surgical orthodontic procedures (Video cephalometrics). Visualization of the facial changes by the patient and clinician is enhanced, alternate treatment plans are evaluated with ease, clinician and patient communication is enhanced, and more realistic patient expectations may be achieved.
5. Three-dimensional computer technology for planning and predicting orthognathic surgery.

CEPHALOGRAMS AS TREATMENT PREDICTION TOOL

Manually treatment prediction is done by two ways:

1. Template method.
2. Tracing overlay method [2].

Variations in the amount of tooth movement can be produced by variations in orthodontic technique and this must be kept in mind when the prediction is being prepared. The prediction procedure can give valuable information about the orthodontic mechanotherapy as well as surgical treatment by establishing exactly where the teeth should be positioned.

Template Method

The use of templates for intermediate tracings between the original and final prediction tracings is mandatory when the maxilla will be repositioned vertically; very helpful when major movements of the teeth must be simulated or when the chin is repositioned; and quite possible when only the mandible is being moved. Thus templates can be moved for any type of prediction. The only reason for not employing this method is that it is more time consuming to prepare a template than to proceed directly to a finished prediction tracing, as is done with the overlay method in uncomplicated mandibular surgery.

The steps in preparing templates for ***maxillary surgery*** in a patient who has crowded lower incisors are shown in Figures 40-46 [2]:

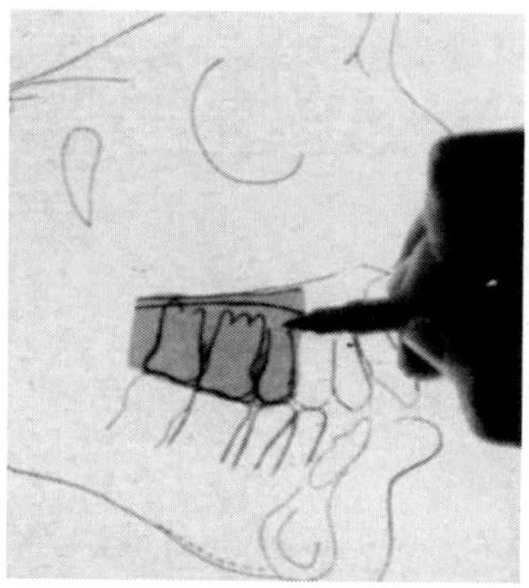

Figure 40. Prepare the maxillary templates by tracing the posterior segment and similarly tracing the maxillary anterior segment.

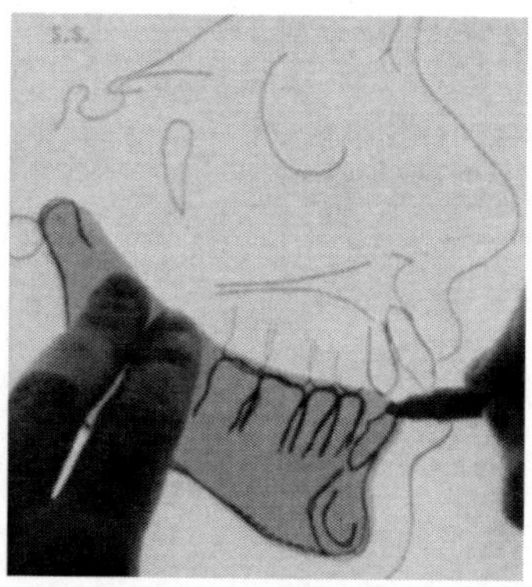

Figure 41. Prepare 2 mandibular templates, one with the crowding resolved without extraction (the incisors must be advanced slightly), and one with extraction (the incisors retracted).

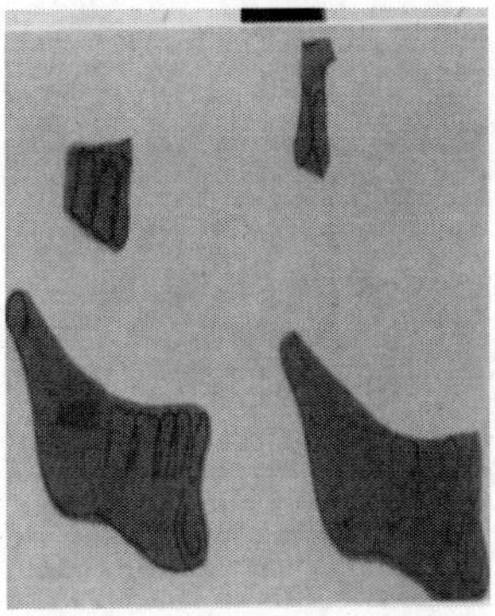

Figure 42. The 4 templates ready for use.

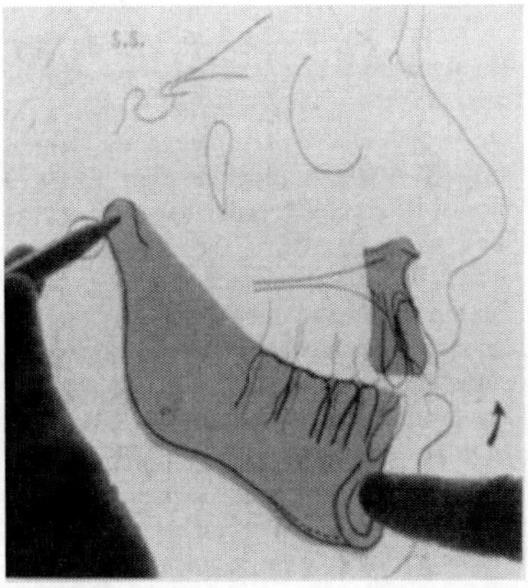

Figure 43. Place the maxillary anterior template in approximately the desired position, about 2mm below the lip line and in approximately the original antero-posterior position. When the nonextraction template is rotated up to the anterior maxillary template, the relationship is not good. Either the maxiallry template should be placed too far forward or there is tendency for anterior cross bite.

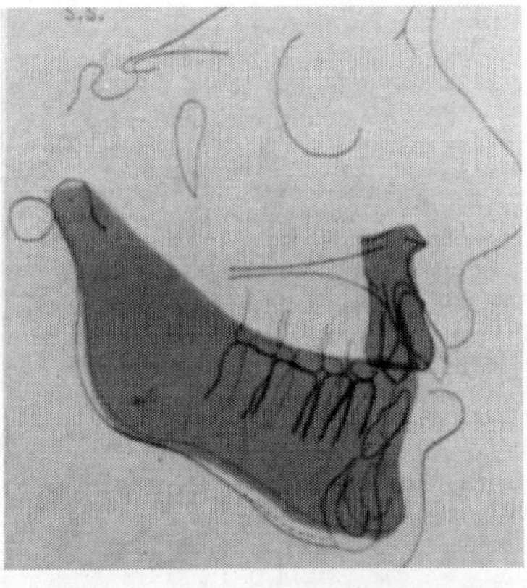

Figure 44. When the extraction template is rotated up to the anterior maxillary template the teeth fit nicely. It is clear that the prominence of the upper anterior teeth will be a function of how much the mandibular incisors are retracted and how far up the maxilla is moved.

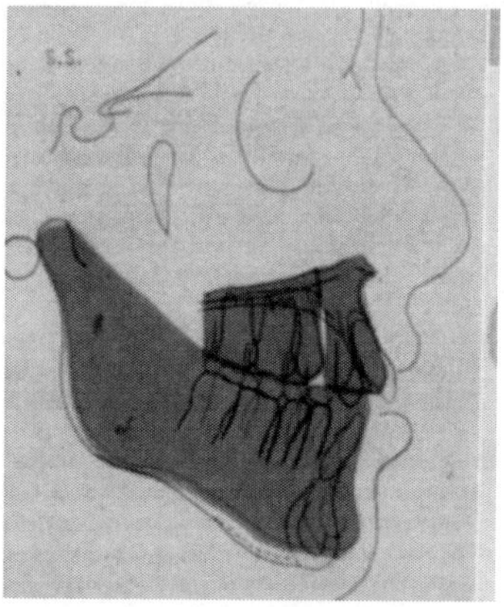

Figure 45. Position of the maxillary posterior template.

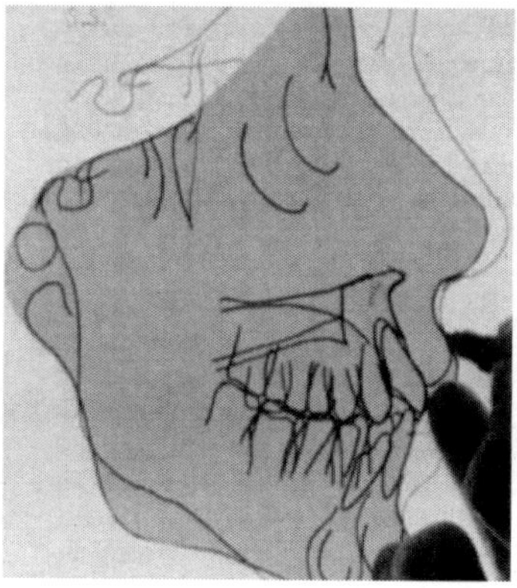

Figure 46. With a clean sheet of tracing paper over the original and the templates, complete the prediction tracing.

Then using following guidelines soft tissue outline is completed (Table 12) [2]:

Table 12. Guidelines of Soft Tissue Outline

Treatment	Soft tissue change
Anteroposterior movement of incisors: Maxillary or mandibular, forward or backward, surgical or orthodontic	60 to 70% of incisor movement
Vertical movement of incisors	Minimal unless jaw rotates
Mandibular advancement	Soft tissue chin 1:1 with bone. Lower lip 60 - 70% with incisor.
Maxillary advancement	Nose: slight elevation of tip Base of upper lip: 20% of pt. A. Upper lip: 60% of incisor protraction, shortens 1-2mm.
Mandibular setback	Chin 1: 1 Lip: 60%
Maxillary setback	Nose: No effect Base of upper lip: 20% of pt. A. Upper lip: 60% of incisor.

Treatment	Soft tissue change
Mandibular setback plus maxillary advancement	Changes similar to a combination of procedures separately.
Maxillary superior repositioning	Nose: widening of alar base. Upper Lip: shortens 1 - 2mm Lower lip: rotates 1:1 with mandible.
Mandibular Advancement plus maxillary superior repositioning	Chin: 1 : 1 Lower lip: 70% of incisors. Upper lip: shortens 1-2 mm. Nose: slight elevation of tip.
Mandibular inferior border repositioning	Soft tissue forward: 60-70% Chin: Up - 1 : 1 with bone Back: 50% with bone Laterally 60% of the bone.

Tracing Overlay Method

This is the simplest way to simulate the effects of mandibular surgery. This method is limited to surgery that does not affect the vertical position of the maxilla (where mandible does not need to rotate around the condyle axis). The steps in preparing prediction tracing in this way are illustrated below in Figures 47 to 52 [2]:

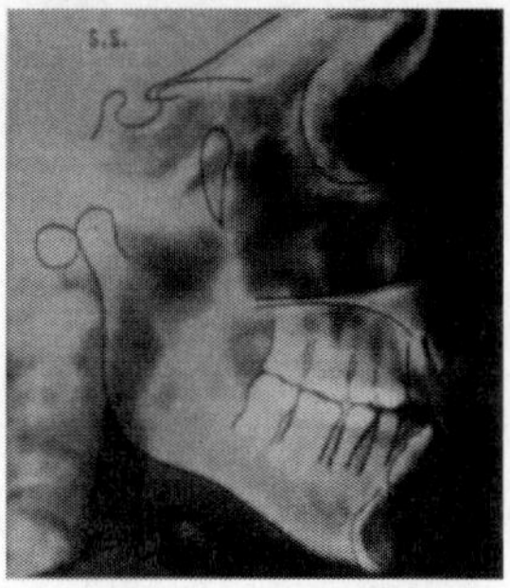

Figure 47. Trace the film, being sure to include all the teeth.

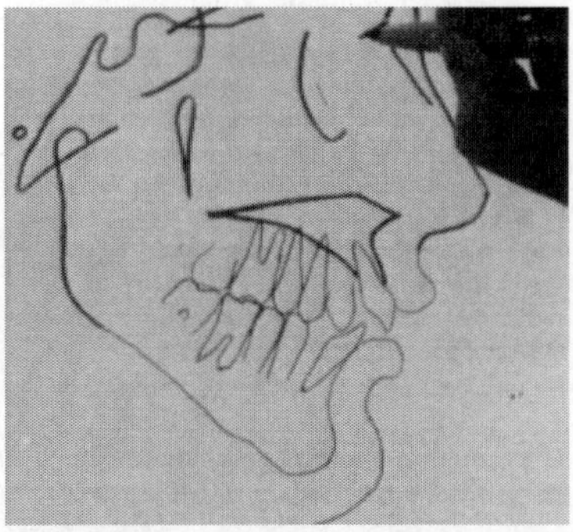

Figure 48. With a new sheet of tracing paper over the original tracing, trace the structures that will not be changed by mandibular surgery: the cranial base, maxilla, and maxillary teeth, mandibular teeth down to the angle, and soft tissue profile down to the base of the nose. Do not trace the mandible or the soft tissue below the nose.

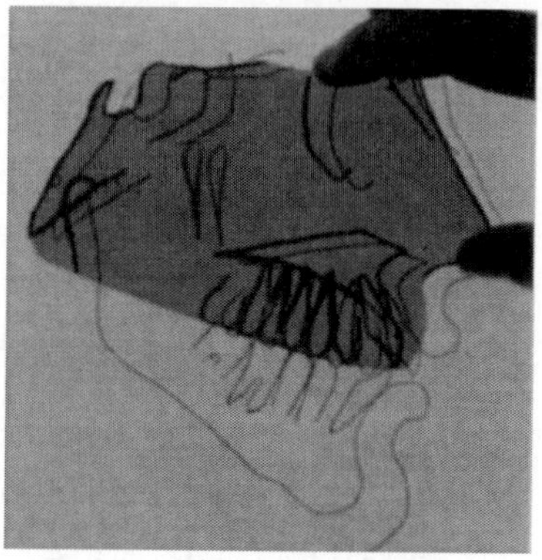

Figure 49. Slide the overlay tracing so that mandibular teeth can be seen through it in their desired post surgical position and trace the lower teeth and jaw.

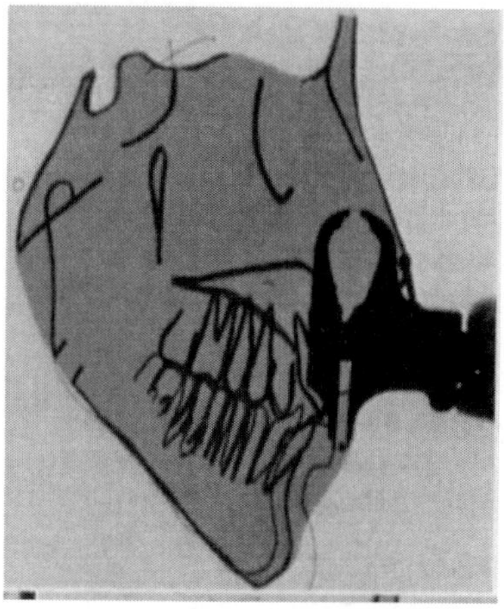

Figure 50. Superimpose the overlay tracing back on the cranial base and measure how far the lower incisor moved forward. The lower lip will go forward two thirds as far. Make a mark that distance forward of the lip.

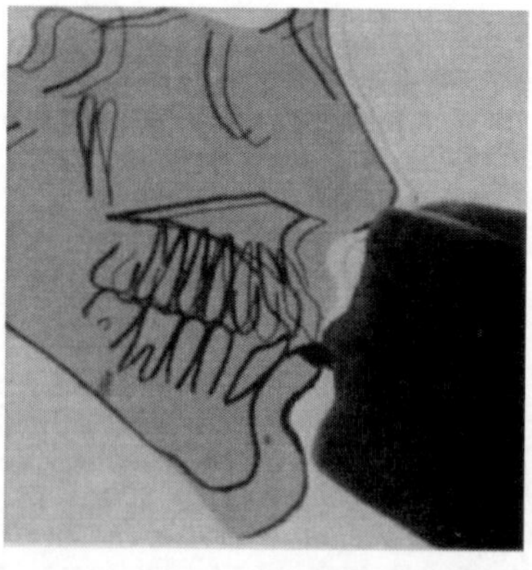

Figure 51. Superimpose again on the mandible. Draw in the soft tissue chin and complete the lower lip outline through the marked point.

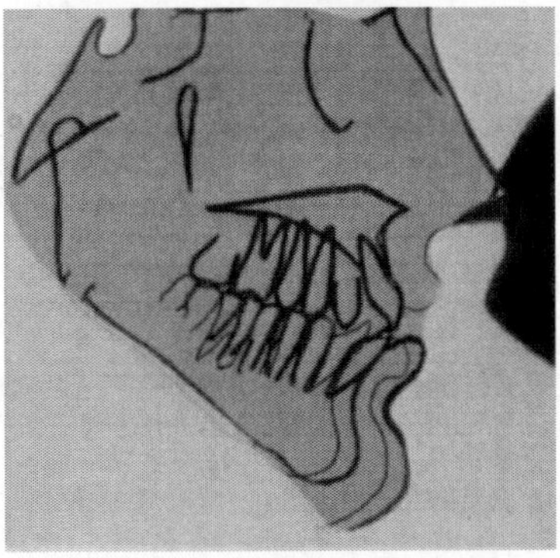

Figure 52. Superimpose again on the cranial base. Complete the soft tissue.

This completes the prediction tracing.

ORTHODONTIC- SURGICAL PREDICTION TRACINGS

As given by EPKER and FISH [40]

I. Cephalometric Prediction Tracing for Mandibular Advancements

The basic reasons for doing predictions for isolated mandibular surgery (advancement or set-back) are:

1. To accurately assess the profile esthetic results which will result from the proposed surgery,
2. To consider the desirability of simultaneous adjunctive procedures such as genioplasty, suprahyoidmyotomy, etc.
3. To help determine the sequencing of surgery and orthodontics (i.e., if the surgery is done first will it be more difficult or easier to do the indicated orthodontics),
4. To help decide what type of orthodontics might best be employed (i.e., extraction versus non-extraction) and
5. To determine the anchorage requirements should extraction treatment be chosen.

Step 1 - Trace the Stable Structures

The first step in producing a prediction tracing is to overlay a piece of acetate paper on the original cephalometric tracing and trace all structures which will not be significantly altered by the surgery and/or orthodontics. For mandibular surgery, these structures will include the deep cranial features, the maxilla, the maxillary occlusal plane, the mandibular ramus and the profile to the base of the nose. Draw in Frankfort Horizontal and a line from nasion to indicate the optimum facial depth, i.e., 89° in females, 90° in males. (Figure 53)

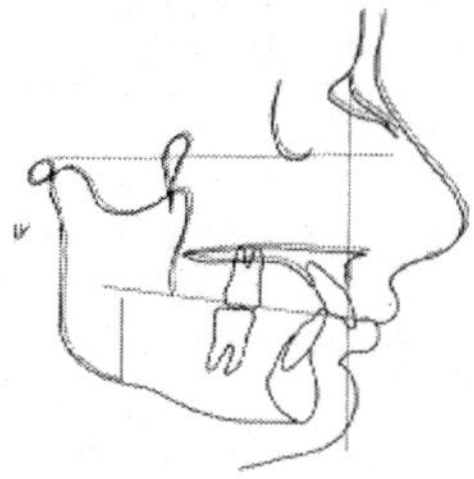

Figure 53. Tracing of stable structures.

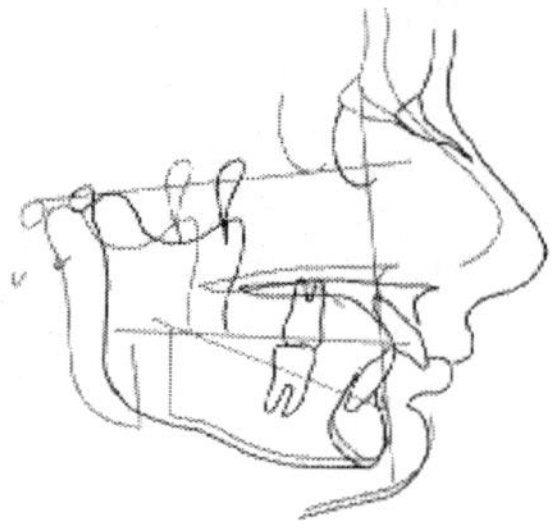

Figure 54. Tracing with changed skeletal structures.

Step 2 - Add Skeletal Portion Changed by Surgery

Slide the prediction tracing to the left and rotate it slightly to position bony pogonion at the optimum facial depth, keeping the mandibular occlusal plane in proper relation to the maxillary occlusal plane. Once a satisfactory position is achieved, trace the distal portion of the mandible, the corpus axis, and the soft tissue chin in this position. There is little change in soft tissue chin thickness, so the soft tissue chin may be drawn in just as it was originally. However, this is so only if the original cephalometric radiograph is taken with the lips in repose. (Figure 54)

Step 3 - New A-Po Line

Construct a new line from Point A to pogonion. If a genioplasty is to be included in the procedure, the anterior portion of this altered chin, be it bone or alloplast, is now constructed to be pogonion for purposes of placing the teeth. (Figure 55)

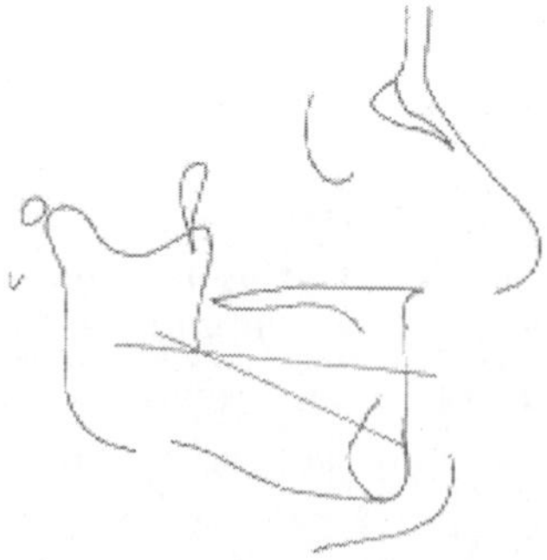

Figure 55. New A-Po Line.

Step 4 - Placing the Teeth

First the lower incisor is placed in its optimum position 1 millimeter ahead of the A-Po line, 1 millimeter above the occlusal plane, and at 22 degrees to the A-Po line.

Old and new mandibles are then superimposed on Corpus Axis at PM and the change in lower incisor position is noted. Arithmetically adding twice this change to the crowding already present allows calculation of the arch length deficiency or excess. Thus, the anterior-posterior position of the lower first molar can be determined and the molar is traced in this position.

The upper first molar is then placed in the desired occlusion and the upper incisor is likewise placed in the optimum position with its long axis 5 degrees more upright than the new facial axis (Figure 56).

Step 5 - Tracing the New Lip Contours

Once the teeth are placed, the lip contours are traced to correspond to the new incisor positions. Very little change in lip thickness is expected, because the original film was taken with the lips in repose.

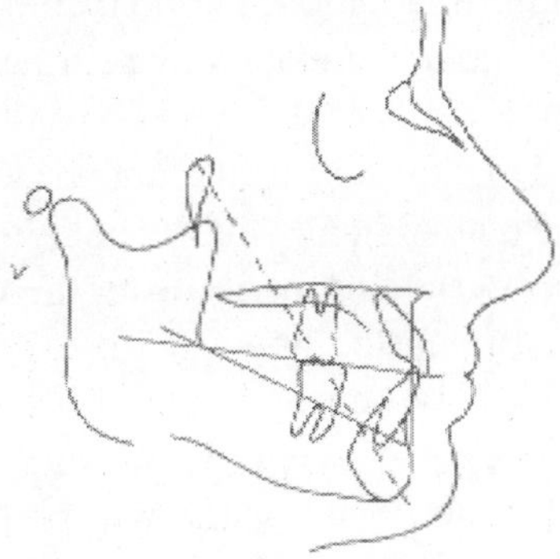

Figure 56. Placing the teeth.

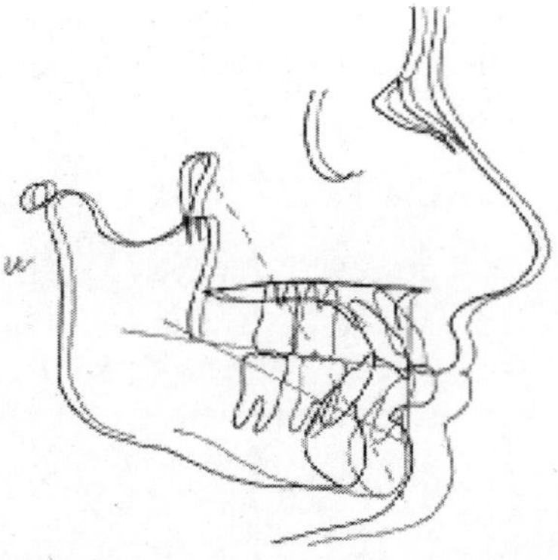

Figure 57. Tracing the new lip contours.

Once completed, the prediction tracing must be viewed as a goal toward which one is working. If the completed tracing represents what you believe is an optimum result, then all is well. However, if there is something that you do not like about it, i.e., chin contour poor, lips too protrusive or too recessive, then the prediction tracing should be modified to correct this problem. Once the prediction tracing is as you like it, the prediction tracing can be superimposed upon the original tracings, registering on the structures not significantly altered by the surgery and/or orthodontics, and the previously stated five basic reasons to do prediction tracings for mandibular surgery can be deliberately and intelligently assessed. (Figure 57)

II. Cephalometric Prediction for Maxillary Superior Repositioning

It is even more important to do prediction tracings for maxillary surgery cases, especially when the primary direction of movement is vertical, to ascertain the effects of the prescribed surgery on the mandible. Specifically, the mandible may require simultaneous surgical repositioning, and by doing the prediction tracing a deliberate decision as to what if anything must be done with it can be made. In addition, the prediction tracing permits one to answer the same basic questions as discussed under mandibular surgery.

Typical Long Face Syndrome patient has narrow alar bases, a long lower third face, excessive interlabial gap, excessive exposure of the upper incisor teeth, a "gummy" smile, a dorsal nasal hump, an obtuse nasolabial angle and a contour-deficient chin. The decision to superiorly reposition the maxilla is made primarily from these esthetic features. The amount of superior repositioning is based upon the upper tooth to lip measurement which is made clinically. Still, we need to know if the maxilla should be moved posteriorly or anteriorly along with the upward movement and we need to know what orthodontics will be necessary. Furthermore, we need to know if autorotation alone will produce an adequate chin or if we will wish to add a genioplasty or consider simultaneous mandibular advancement. These questions can be answered from a prediction tracing.

Step 1 - Trace the Stable Structures

As is the case with all prediction tracings, we again begin by tracing the structures which will not be modified either surgically or orthodontically. This should include point A (Figure 58).

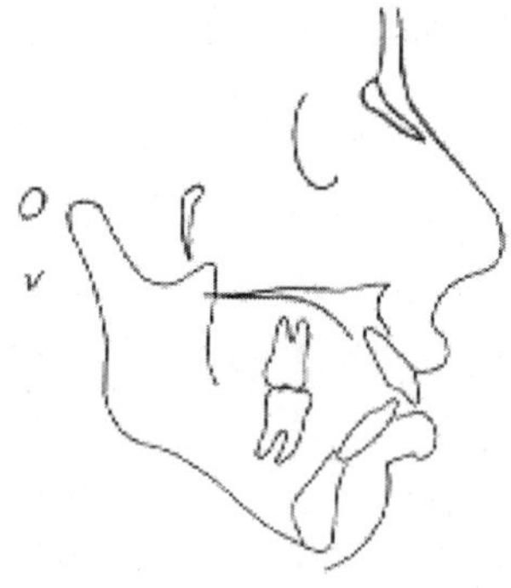

Figure 58. Tracing of stable structures.

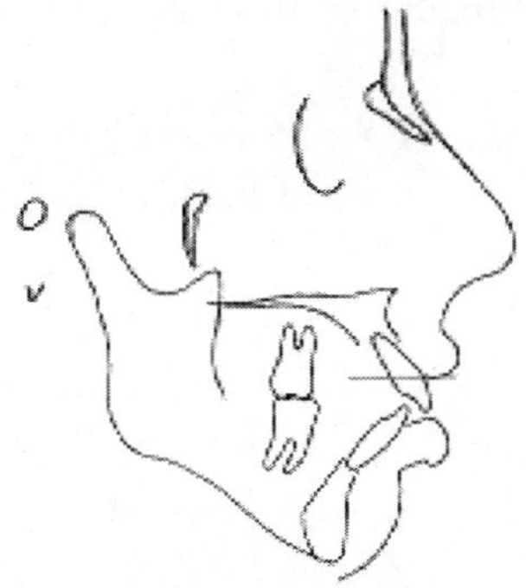

Figure 59. Determination of Ideal Vertical Position for the Upper Incisor.

Step 2 - Determination of Ideal Vertical Position for the Upper Incisor

Regardless of how accurate your cephalometric technique, we recommend that the measurement of the amount of upper central incisor exposed, i.e., that from stomion of the upper lip to incisal edge, be made clinically with the patient standing in a relaxed posture. This is the single most important measurement in preparation for superior repositioning of the maxilla and can be confirmed cephalometrically. Once the amount of incisor exposed beneath the upper lip is determined, the "ideal" amount of superior repositioning of the upper incisor can be determined by the formula:

$$X = y - 2/0.8$$

where X is the amount of superior repositioning necessary and Y is the amount of upper incisor showing. This formula is used because the upper lip tends to shorten approximately 20% of the amount of superior surgical repositioning; thus, a 1:1 relationship between the amount of tooth showing and the amount of repositioning necessary does not exist. Furthermore, if the superior movement is to be accompanied by posterior movement of the incisors and an acute nasolabial angle is present, the lip will not shorten quite as much as predicted. Conversely, with an obtuse nasolabial angle and anterior movement of the incisor, the lip will tend to shorten slightly more. These slight variations may be disregarded, unless the anterior-posterior change is more than 6 millimeters.

Once the desired amount of vertical incisor repositioning is determined, draw a line parallel to Frankfort horizontal on the prediction tracing to represent the desired vertical position. (Figure 59)

Step 3 - Autorotation of the Mandible

Superimpose the original and prediction tracings and, keeping the mandibular condyle in the same position, rotate the prediction tracing clockwise until the occlusal plane is 1 mm above the line indicating the desired position of the upper incisor. A no of studies have been carried out to discover a true centre of mandibular rotation [41, 42]. Although the results are variable, the centre of rotation appears to be posterior and inferior to the condyle in mastoid region. But as a practical matter location of centre of rotation makes little difference in predicting the final position of mandible and bests result come when using centre of condyle as centre of rotation [2]. Trace the mandible in this position. The corpus axis and the occlusal plane are also traced in at this time.

The change in point A and the soft tissue chin contour must be carefully studied at this time. To allow easier observation of these features, one may wish to trace, with dotted lines, the soft tissue chin, the lower incisor, and Point A.

The first feature that must be noted is the change in Point A. If this point moves posteriorly as it often will in order to correct an existing Class II occlusion, we then use old Point A in determining the A-Po relationship for the lower incisor. This point is frequently obliterated by the surgery and furthermore the soft tissues of the midface, relatively unaffected by the surgery, still retain the same basic relationship with old Point A making the physiologic basis for the A-Po line valid while using the old Point A. Conversely, if point A moves anteriorly the soft tissue will be moved forward and the new Point A is used to construct the A-Po line. (Figure 60)

Step 4 - Genioplasty Determination

The second feature which must be noted is the new soft tissue chin position. If the chin is adequate, then genioplasty is not necessary. However, if the chin is still weak, either mandibular advancement or some type of genioplasty must be added to the treatment plan for optimum esthetics. Conversely, if the chin is too strong, then some procedure to reduce it may be required. Ideally, we would like to determine the "normal" position for the soft tissue chin and then plan our genioplasty to produce this desired result. For bony genioplasties, the ratio of anterior-posterior soft tissue change to bony change is about 0.6:1, thus, if 5 millimeters more chin is desired, a bony advancement of 8 millimeters will be required. If alloplastic material is to be added, this ratio approaches 1:1 thus 5 millimeters of alloplast will produce 5 millimeters more soft tissue chin.

For patients who are not to undergo orthodontic treatment or where the lower incisors cannot be retracted sufficiently, best chin-lip-nose balance is usually attained by placing an alloplastic genioplasty thick enough to bring the material to a line from Point A and passing 1 to 3 millimeters lingual to the lower incisor tip, thus producing a "normal" A-Po relationship for the lower incisor. Once the amount of genioplasty has been determined, the new A-Po line can be constructed using the genioplasty as a new pognonion and either the old Point A or new Point A as discussed previously.

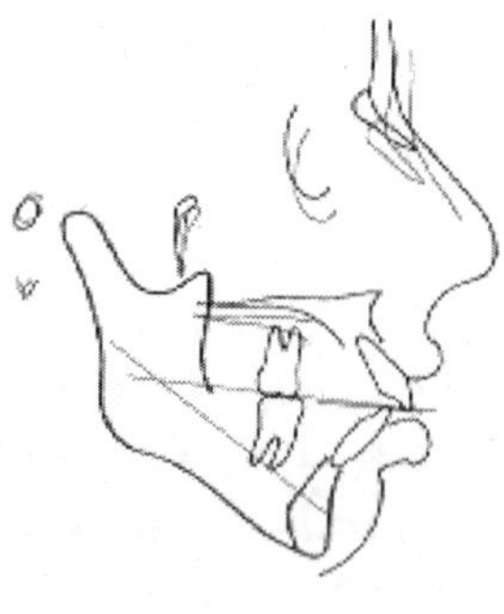

Figure 60. Autorotation of the Mandible.

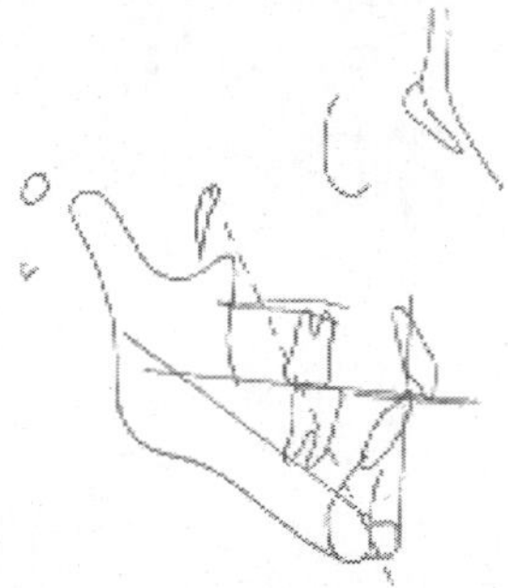

Figure 61. Placement of teeth in ideal positions.

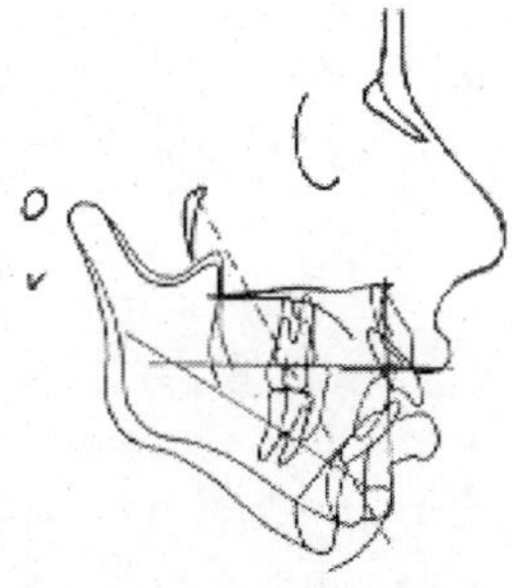

Figure 62. Nasal Outline.

Step 5 - Placement of Teeth In Ideal Positions

After placing the teeth in their ideal position trace the new profile. (Figure 61)

Step 6 - Nasal Outline

With superior repositioning of the maxilla, the nasal tip is generally elevated slightly. This is more pronounced if the maxilla is moved upward and forward, less pronounced if upward and backward. The lower border of the nose is relatively unchanged though it too may be elevated a small amount. Accordingly, the prediction tracing should be placed on the original with the fixed landmarks superimposed and the nasal outline traced with the aforementioned alterations. (Figure 62)

Step 7 - Upper Lip

The upper lip reacts to superior repositioning in the following ways: 1) the length from subnasale to upper lip stomion shortens 1/5 of the amount of superior repositioning, 2) the thickness increases by 1/3 of the amount of incisor retraction, and 3) the lip thins out slightly if the upper incisor is moved forward, but in all but the most extreme instances this is unnoticeable. To trace the new upper lip one should superimpose on the fixed cranial structures and study the change in incisor position.

If the upper incisor is retracted such that it lies posterior to an imaginary line from the labial surface to Point A on the original tracing, then lip support has been reduced and one should trace the new lip in the following manner:

Divide the vertical distance from old incisor tip to new incisor tip into fifths and the anterior-posterior distance into thirds. Move the prediction tracing down 1/5 and forward 2/3 and draw in the new lip vermillion. Connect the new lip vermillion to the previously traced subnasale in an artistic manner. Subnasale is affected so little by superior repositioning that for prediction it can be considered a fixed point.

If the upper incisor has moved directly up the line from the labial surface to Point A of the original tracing, then lip support is unchanged and one should trace the new lip in the following manner:

Divide the vertical distance from old incisor tip to new incisor tip into fifths. Move the prediction tracing down 1/5 and trace the new lip, connecting it to subnasale as above.

If, the upper incisor is forward of the line from labial surface to Point A of the original tracing, then lip support has been increased and the new lip is traced as follows:

Divide the vertical distance from old incisor tip to new incisor tip into fifths. Move the prediction tracing down 1/5. Then, while maintaining this vertical position, rotate and slide the prediction tracing such that the long axis of the upper incisor in the prediction tracing is parallel to, and the labial surface is flush with, the line from the labial surface to Point A of the original tracing. Trace the new lip in this position. This effectively maintains the original lip thickness. (Figure 63)

Step 8 - Lower Lip

In most instances the lower lip vermillion is traced in the same relation to the lower incisors as existed prior to treatment. Superimpose the lower incisor on the prediction tracing over that on the original and trace the lower lip.

Where the lower incisors are retracted 5 millimeters or more, we find that the lip tends to thicken slightly. Thus the lower incisors are not exactly superimposed, but the prediction tracing is moved slightly to the lingual of an exact superimposition (i.e., the lip thickens slightly) and the lip traced in this position. Some artistic freedom must be employed when dealing with a hypotonic lip. In our experience, the hypotonic lip may increase mildly in tonicity following production of lip competence and added support for the lip via augmentation genioplasty. If one feels that such a result is likely, then the lip would be traced slightly thinner for purposes of prediction (Figure 64).

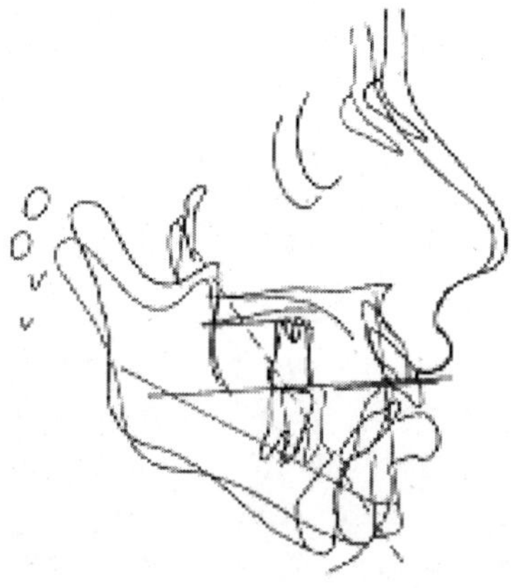

Figure 63. Tracing of Upper Lip.

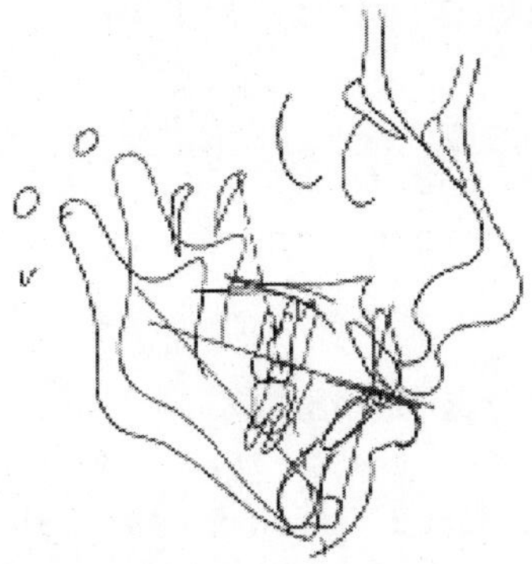

Figure 64. Tracing of Lower Lip.

Step 9 - Chin

If no genioplasty is projected, the soft tissue chin will be relatively unaffected by treatment and should be traced by simply superimposing on the mandibular symphysis. If a sliding genioplasty is done, the chin is traced by first superimposing on the original symphysis and then sliding the prediction tracing back 6/10 of the amount of the genioplasty and tracing the new chin contour. If an alloplastic implant is added, the new chin contour can be determined by simply superimposing the alloplastic implant on the original symphysis and tracing the chin.

Once the tracing is completed, we again must study it to determine if indeed we have achieved a satisfactory result. To once again gain optimum appreciation for the proposed changes superimposition of the original and prediction tracing is done frequently, it is necessary to do several prediction tracings, trying different surgical approaches to a problem (i.e., superior repositioning vs. superior repositioning with genioplasty vs. superior repositioning with mandibular advancement) before one can determine which result is best. Certainly it is better to retreat a patient on paper than to wish that a different surgical approach had been employed after the fact. (Figure 65)

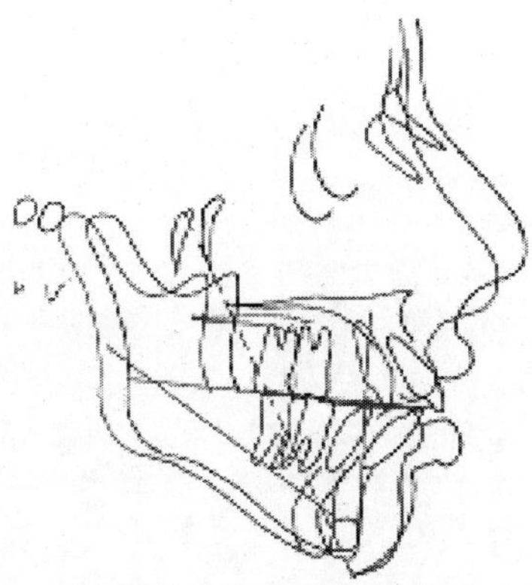

Figure 65. Tracing of Chin.

III. Cephalometric Prediction Tracing for Combined Maxillary and Mandibular Cases

The basic technique involved is to trace the stable structures, place the maxilla in the desired position both vertically and anterior-posteriorly and then place the mandible in its desired position.

Step 1 - Trace the Stable Structures (Figure 66)

Step 2 - Determine the Ideal Vertical Position for the Upper Incisor

Some care must be taken here, as the use of the aforementioned formula may not be entirely accurate. In the patient with an obtuse nasolabial angle, where the maxilla will come forward to increase lip support, slightly more shortening of the lip will be produced than might otherwise be expected. Thus, slightly more superior movement of the incisor will be desirable. Superimpose the original and the prediction tracings and draw a line parallel with Frankfort horizontal to indicate the desired vertical position of the upper incisor. Trace a line from original point A tangent to the labial of the upper incisor as a reference for the original upper lip support. (Figure 67)

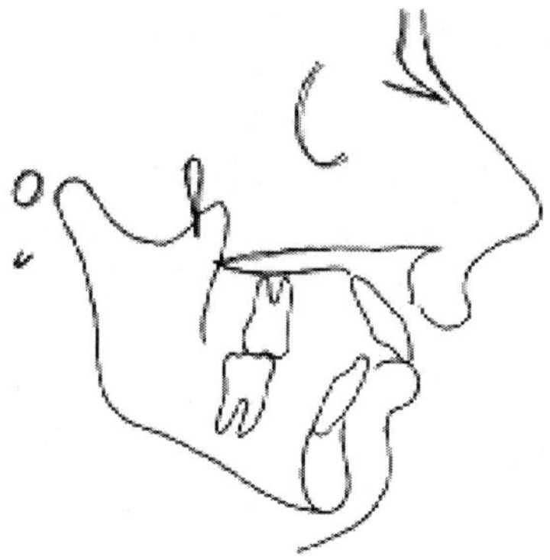

Figure 66. Tracing of stable structures.

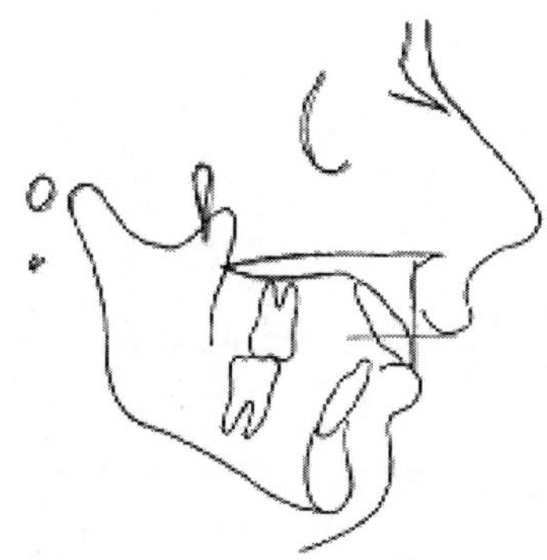

Figure 67. Determination of Ideal Vertical Position for the Upper Incisor.

Step 3 - Autorotation of the Occlusal Plane

Keeping the condyle in the same position, rotate the prediction tracing clockwise until the occlusal plane is 1mm above the line indicating the desired position of the upper incisor. Trace the occlusal plane and the mandibular ramus in this position.

Without moving the drawings, one should now assess the anterior-posterior change of the maxilla by such rotation. This is done by comparing the new Point A-incisor line to the one made to show the position prior to rotation. Frequently, enough anterior movement has been effected by the rotation alone and the anterior maxilla can be traced at this point. If, however, more anterior movement is desired, then the maxilla is moved anteriorly along the occlusal plane by sliding the tracing posteriorly until the desired amount of forward movement (i.e., increase in lip support) is attained.

With the desired anterior-posterior maxillary position attained, point A should be drawn in. The upper incisor and molar position are marked for future reference. By adding Frankfort Horizontal and the optimum facial depth line we now have a tracing which should look like that made of the fixed skeletal landmarks drawn in the first step of the mandibular advancement procedure, except that the nose has not yet been traced. (Figure 68)

Step 4 - Mandibular Movement

This is done exactly as was done in Step 2 under mandibular advancement. (Figure 69)

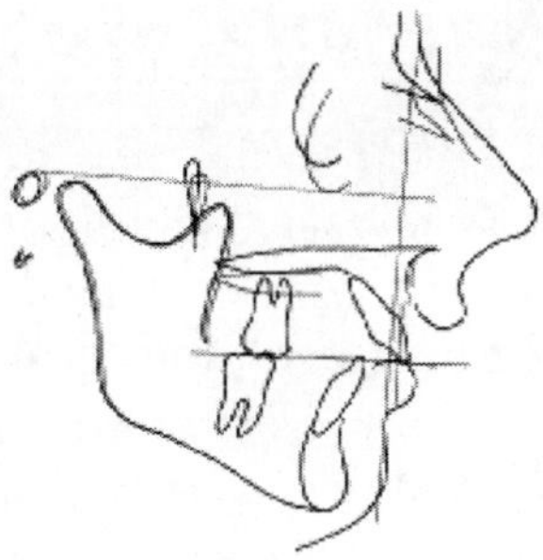

Figure 68. Autorotation of the Occlusal Plane.

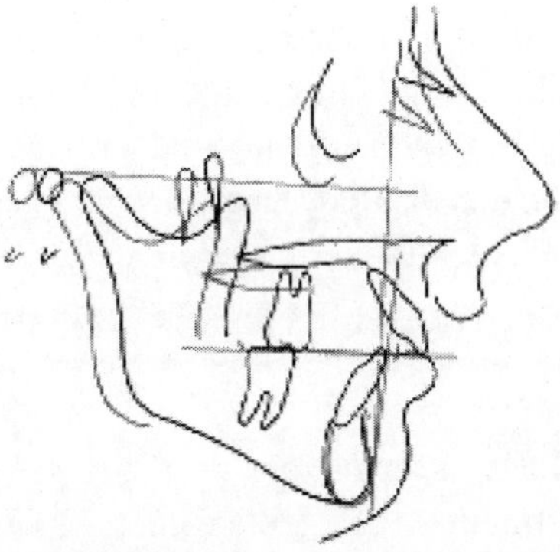

Figure 69. Tracing of Mandibular Movement.

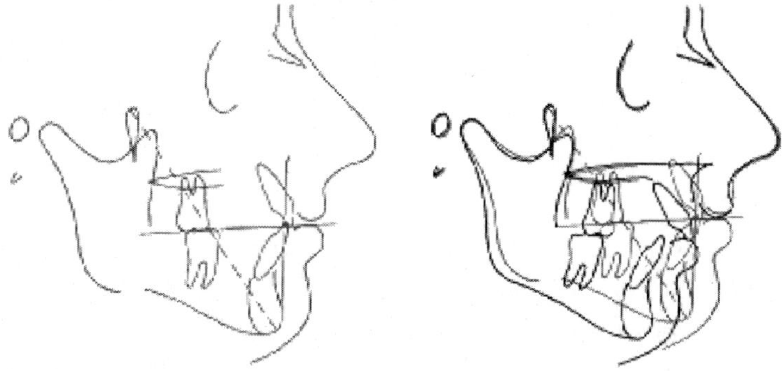

Figure 70. Completing the Tracing.

Steps 5-10 - Completing the Tracing

Once the new position of the mandible has been traced, the balance of the tracing is done as outlined in Steps 4-9 under Maxillary Superior Repositioning. (Figure 70)

Prediction Tracings Using TOMAC

TOMAC is a unique surgical-orthodontic treatment planning system given by Tony McCollum (hence name TOMAC) in which VTO is constructed in three stages: test, presurgical-orthodontic, and surgical [43]. The essential underlying principle is that the soft-tissue profile is changed first, setting a goal toward which hard-tissue changes are adapted.

Test VTO

This is where the various orthodontic and surgical options are tested and the optimum combination is visualized. In the anteroposterior plane, the facial contour angle (FCA) is changed to the chosen ideal. The upper and lower jaws, or both, are traced in their new positions according to the soft-tissue reactions to surgical movements, and the teeth are then decompensated accordingly. The incisor movements are measured and reconciled with arch-length discrepancies and with the physiological positions of the teeth in the alveolar bone.

In the vertical plane, the key is the position of the maxillary incisor in relation to the relaxed upper lip. The maxillary incisors are moved vertically on the tracing, if necessary, into their ideal positions relative to the upper lip, and the mandible is autorotated so that the correct vertical relationship of the maxillary and mandibular incisors is obtained. The new FCA is measured and compared with the chosen ideal FCA. Appropriate anteroposterior jaw movements are then effected to obtain the ideal total profile. The teeth are decompensated into positions most favorable to the desired surgical changes, keeping in mind arch-length discrepancies and physiological positions in the alveolar bone. The incisor movements required to accomplish the skeletal changes are measured for use in the presurgical VTO.

Presurgical-Orthodontic VTO

This is constructed from the information in the test VTO. Any necessary incisor decompensations, molar adjustments, and soft-tissue changes become the orthodontic objectives prior to the surgical procedure.

Surgical VTO

The surgical VTO is constructed over the presurgical VTO, with the surgical cuts diagramed on the tracings of the jaws. The simulated surgical movements are governed by the decompensated positions of the incisors. The soft-tissue profile is then drawn according to the expected soft-tissue/hard-tissue ratios of movement.

Prediction Tracing for Mandibular Advancement

Following steps are performed to construct the VTO for mandibular advancement. For a mandibular setback, the directions would be reversed.

Test VTO

1. Overlay a new acetate sheet on the original tracing. Trace in the hard tissues that will not change with surgery: anterior cranial base, the maxilla, the maxillary molars and incisors, and the proximal segment of the mandible and the soft-tissue outline from glabella to subnasale draw in the upper facial contour plane, and construct the lower facial contour plane at the ideal angulation (8° to 11°). Add the occlusal plane.
2. Superimpose the tracing on the occlusal plane, and slide the tracing to the left to simulate mandibular advancement (or to the right for a mandibular setback) so that the soft-tissue chin is tangent to the new, ideal lower facial contour plane. The basic landmarks of the profile: upper face (glabella), midface (subnasale), and lower face (pogonion) will now approximate normal positions. Draw in the symphysis, the distal segment of the mandible, and the mandibular molars and incisors (this is before any orthodontic movement.) The maximum surgical movement that can be achieved is 6-8mm with a mandibular advancement and 6mm with a mandibular reduction. There are exceptions, but these extreme cases should be discussed with the surgeon.

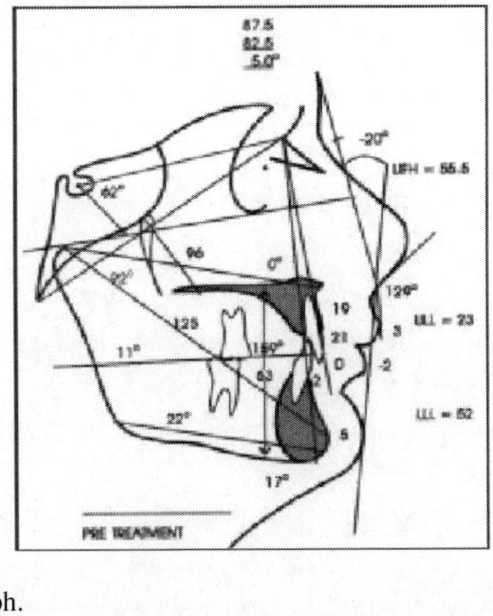

Figure 71. Original Radiograph.

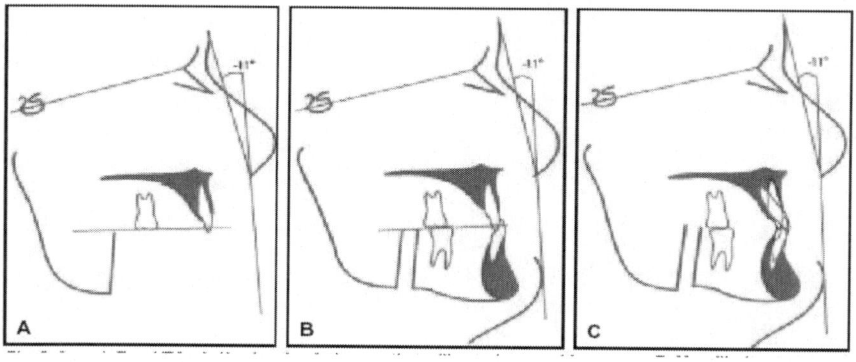

Figure 72. A. Hard and soft tissues that will not change with surgery. B. Mandibular structures after advancement. C. Incisor decompensation needed to achieve best profile.

3. Reconcile the incisor movements or decompensation required to create the ideal profile with arch length and the bony anatomy Make any extraction decisions as necessary, and evaluate the anchorage requirements. If a normal interincisal relationship with the teeth in good physiological position in the alveolar bone cannot be achieved, compromise profiles will have to be sought. Thus, the optimum combination of orthodontic and surgical movements required for the best possible profile is determined. The information derived from the test VTO is applied in the orthodontic and surgical VTOs that follow. (Figure 71, 72)

Presurgical-Orthodontic VTO

Construct a new VTO to reflect the orthodontic movements that will be needed to allow surgery to create the ideal (or nearest to ideal) profile. Bite opening or closing is measured by the change in angulation of the line from condylion to gnathion. It is important to draw in the soft-tissue changes that will occur as a result of any orthodontic decompensation. (Figure 73)

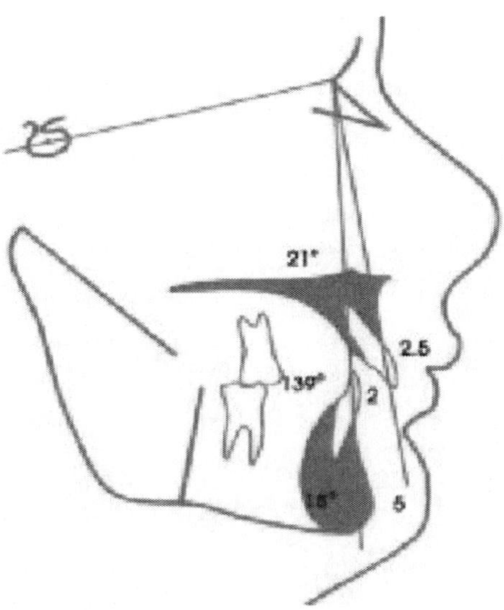

Figure 73. Presurgical-orthodontic VTO.

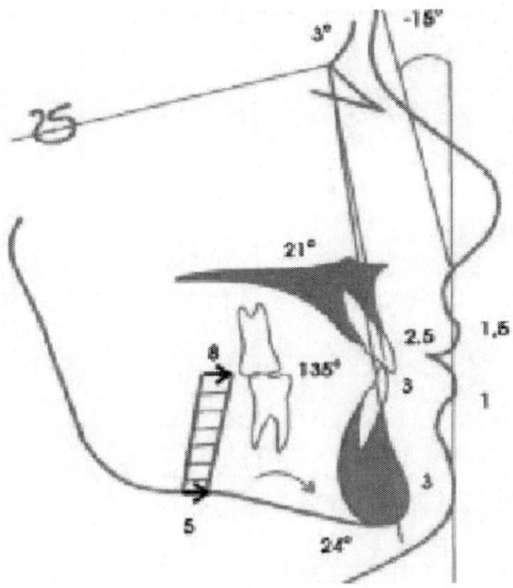

Figure 74. Surgical VTO.

Surgical VTO

1. Place a new acetate sheet over the surgical-orthodontic VTO. Trace in the hard tissues that will not change with surgery and the soft tissues from glabella to subnasale, including the nose. The proximal and distal segments of the mandible should be separated by an osteotomy cut, represented by a nearly vertical line in the second molar region. Trace in the proximal segment.
2. Advance (or set back) the mandible along the occlusal plane by moving the tracing paper to the left (or right) so that the incisors form a normal Class I relationship. In most cases, the molars should then be Class I as well. In patients where a deep overbite correction is required in surgery, rotate the tracing paper clockwise (an opening rotation of the distal segment) to achieve a Class I incisor relationship. This is a surgically stable maneuver. (Figure 74)
3. Trace in the distal segment of the mandible, the osteotomy cut, the molars, the incisors, and the soft-tissue chin outline. In anteroposterior mandibular surgical repositioning, the soft-tissue chin generally follows the bony chin in a 1:1 ratio, although a mild flattening of the soft tissue is seen in some cases. Measure the distances between the old and new osteotomy cut lines superiorly and inferiorly to establish the amount of mandibular movement.
4. Draw in the lips. Practically speaking, the lower lip advances 75% of the distance of a mandibular incisor advancement, and retracts similarly with mandibular setback.
5. It is now vital to test the chin position for profile harmony. Draw in the new FCA, and compare it to the norm. Measure and evaluate the positions of the lips relative to the lower facial contour plane. If necessary, repeat the VTOs using different orthodontic goals until a satisfactory esthetic result is achieved.

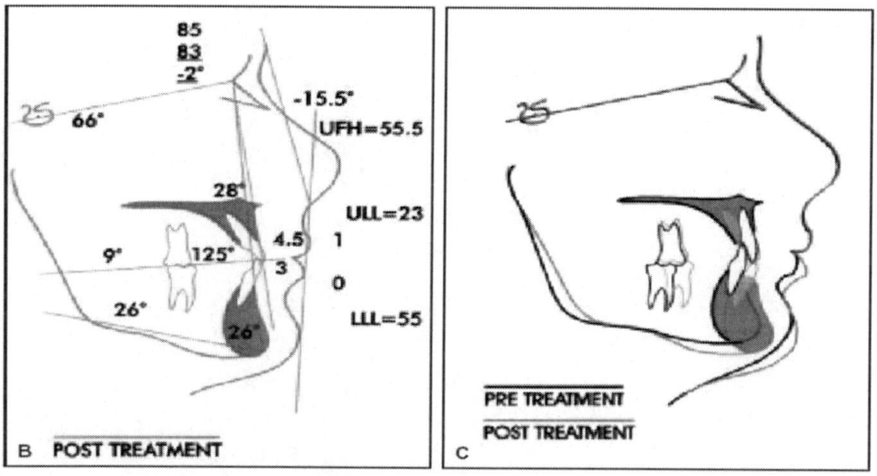

Figure 75. Completed Superimposition with results.

Results

The treatment objectives were achieved. Because a downward and forward movement of the distal segment of the mandible was required to correct the large overjet and deep overbite, the chin was not advanced as much as the target FCA would have indicated. Still, the chin and lips were in favorable balance after treatment. (Figure 75)

Prediction Tracing for Maxillary Excess

The key to planning the correction of maxillary vertical excess, with or without anterior open bite, is that the diagnostic lateral cephalogram must be taken with the lips completely relaxed. The significant soft-tissue measurements are the interlabial gap and the distance from the incisal tip to the upper lip stomion.

On the test VTO, the new maxillary incisor vertical position is represented by a line 2 mm below a tangent to the inferior aspect of the relaxed upper lip. The mandible is rotated about the condylion until the mandibular central incisor is 1-1.5 mm above this horizontal line. When subsequently tracing in the maxilla, it is important that the maxilla not be advanced more than **2 mm** from the original NA line. Further advancement will cause the mandibular incisors to be too proclined and to require uprighting or retroclination. Excessive advancement of the maxilla to match the closing rotation of the mandible can also have undesirable soft-tissue effects, such as excessive shortening of the upper lip, deflection of the nasal tip, and flaring of the nostrils. In all cases, the new facial contour angle (FCA) should be measured to determine whether there are profile discrepancies. (Figure 76, 77)

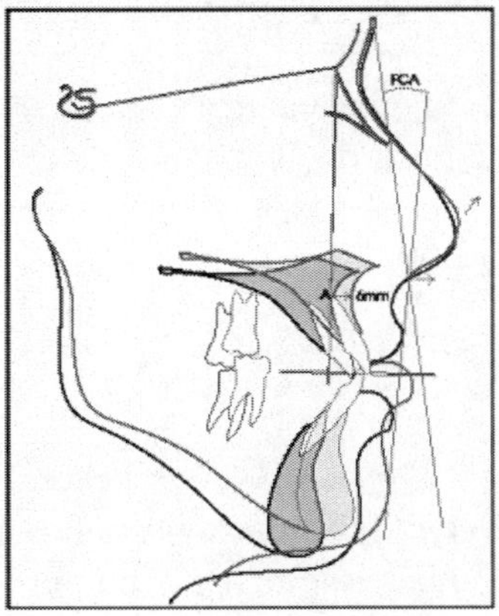

Figure 76. A Point advanced too far (more than 2mm) after autorotation of mandible.

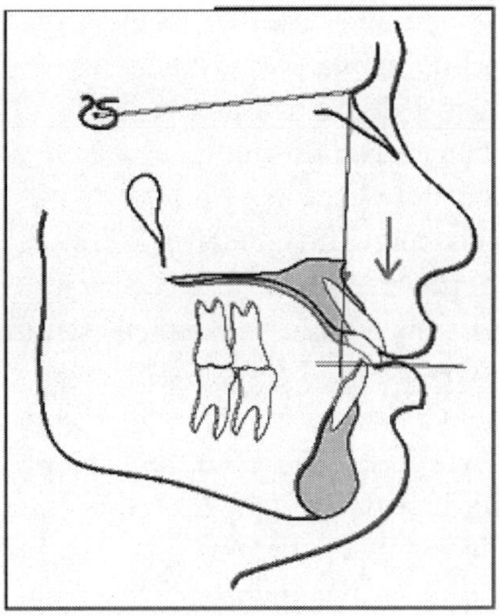

Figure 77. Incisor relationships reassessed after downgraft of maxilla.

Prediction Tracing for Maxillary Vertical Deficiency

In maxillary vertical deficiency, the maxillary incisors are usually underexposed relative to the relaxed upper lip. The new maxillary incisor vertical position is represented on the test VTO by a line 2mm below the relaxed upper lip. An extra 1mm exposure of the maxillary incisor can be budgeted to allow for surgical relapse, since down grafting of the maxilla can be surgically unstable despite improved fixation techniques. The incisor relationships are then assessed and reconciled with arch length and their physiological positions in the bone.

Treatment of Combined Maxillary and Mandibular Deformities

On the test VTO, the vertical discrepancies are corrected first by autorotating the mandible to the desired vertical position, which is determined by elevating the anterior maxilla and maxillary incisors along the NA line. The anteroposterior variations of the soft-tissue profile, facial skeleton, and teeth are then reassessed. The test profile is measured from the FCA.

Three possibilities may occur:

1. *The FCA is within normal limits*. If so, the necessary compensation is assessed by reconciling it with arch-length discrepancies and bony anatomy. If the ideal incisor positions cannot be obtained, the facial contour will be compromised. This is important to know before treatment begins.
2. *The FCA is too acute*. This indicates either that the mandible is too protrusive or the maxilla is retrusive, making it important to reexamine the original diagnosis. If there are signs of maxillary anteroposterior deficiency, then subnasale can be advanced. Remember that soft-tissue subnasale advances at a ratio of 50% of the maxillary surgical movement. Incisor decompensations can be made, taking into account arch-length discrepancies, bony anatomy, and gingival condition. If there is a mandibular excess, then a mandibular setback is required. If the FCA is still too acute or the reverse overjet is 8mm or more, then anteroposterior surgery of both jaws is required in combination with vertical movement. Reduction genioplasties are also useful in obtaining a good profile, but should be balanced with lip structure. The labiomental angle should not be too obtuse, and nasal esthetics must also be considered.
3. *The FCA is too obtuse*. Consideration should be given to mandibular advancement and/or advancement genioplasty, provided the genioplasty is in harmony with the lip positions. Appropriate incisor decompensations will be required. It is seldom necessary to surgically set back the maxilla except in cases of severe bidental protrusion, and this is usually done in the first premolar area.

In some cases where the upper lip is procumbent and the nasolabial angle is acute, it will be necessary to plan for posterior movement of the upper lip. On the test VTO, the upper lip is retracted first, taking into account lip strain, widening of the nasolabial angle, and protrusion relative to the lower facial contour plane. The maxillary incisors will need to be retracted, and decisions made regarding anchorage and extractions. The new overjet is measured, and the ideal Facial Contour Angle is drawn. Any convexity or concavity is then addressed by advancement or setback of the mandible and/or the chin.

Videocephalometrics as Treatment Prediction Tool

With the ever increasing use of orthognathic surgery for the correction of dentofacial deformities, the demands on the planning skills of the orthodontist and the surgeon have increased as well. What surgeons or orthodontists consider ideal may not be the same as patient's desires. Function, esthetics, and shaping the patient's expectations into reality must all be addressed while keeping in mind the patient's best interests and desires [44].

In the past few years, doctors have used adjuncts such as cephalograms, profile tracings and photographs in an attempt to define facial parameters in planning orthognathic surgery cases [45] Acetate tracings are very useful to determine placement of hard tissue and the response of soft tissue to those movements. However, they are of lesser value for visualization of the profile outcome and obviously of virtually no value in frontal prediction. The final esthetic outcome is heavily dependent on the experience and/or artistic skill of the treatment planner [46]. Therefore photograph modification was advocated in the 1980s for improved communication and planning [47], but does not allow the planner to visualize limiting factors such as the dental relationships (overjet) or differential soft tissue reaction to hard tissue movement. Moreover gaps in the manipulated photographs are unavoidable.

With the evolution of computer technology, visualization of coordinated facial and dental plans has been greatly facilitated. Video imaging technology allows the orthodontist to gather frontal and profile images and modify them to project overall esthetic treatment goals. In the case of surgical treatment, patients are very motivated to know what they will look like after surgery. The use of video imaging technology allows us to modify facial images to project treatment goals and then discuss them with the patient [48]. The video image is much more realistic than photograph simulation and it is much easier for the patient to comprehend than just the soft tissue profile of a cephalometric tracing. Video imaging, then, appears to be the next step in the natural progression of the application of technology to orthodontic treatment planning.

The advantage that video cephalometric planning often offers is that: [44]

1. It provides an image from which the patient and surgeon can visualize the aesthetic treatment objectives.
2. It provides the capability to measure calibrated distances and angles on the planning image.
3. It allows quantification of the planned dental and/or osseous movements to reduce the guesswork as to the facial response to our orthodontic treatment plan; and
4. It allows the clinician to test various treatment plans before deciding on the final plan.

However there are certain weaknesses of videoimaging that should be kept in mind: [44]

1. Predictions have same soft tissue uncertainty as hand drawn cephalometric prediction tracings.
2. Possible heightened expectations of the patient beyond what can be realistically achieved can occur.
3. It is very difficult to predict what changes occur in frontal view.
4. Soft tissue changes on profile are always 1:1. there is no way, as yet, to make proportional soft tissue changes.

Hardware Used for Video Imaging

Following hardware allows capturing and manipulation of the patient images [44]:

1. IBM compatible personal computer.
   a. 512K Random Access Memory (RAM) required to run AT&T Truevision Image Processing software.
   b. 640K RAM required to run Orthographics software.
2. Truevision Advanced Raster Graphics Adapter 16 board.
3. An 8087 math co-processor. An analog Red-Green-Blue (RGB) monitor or composite video color monitor.
4. JVC video camera with RGB and composite output.
5. Summagraphics 961 or 1201 graphics tablet.

Software Used for Videoimaging

1. TIPS by AT&T, a graphics software language and allows the personal computer to capture digitized images from the video camera and facilitates modification of the image through its sophisticated drawing and editing features.
2. Orthographics by Mathematica addresses a more specific set of applications for the orthodontist or surgeon as opposed to wide range of applications of TIPS [44].

Videoimaging: The Sequence of Diagnosis and Treatment Planning

Videoimaging and treatment planning has two major phases: counseling and videocephalometric treatment planning [49]. The counseling phase involves the use of facial or dental image modification without any quantitative aspect to the process. It is simply a graphic method of communication. Once the patient decides that he or she does wish to proceed with treatment, partially based on the images projected, the planning phase is then carried out which permits quantification of the treatment plan so that the clinician knows precisely what and how much what he or she plans to do. It involves integration of facial profile image with the cephalometric radiograph.

By having the ability to see where the teeth lie in relation to face, clinicians can make judgement about the changes needed for occlusal correction. In the adult patient, the computer prediction can be quite accurate. In the adult, the major inaccuracy is the actual treatment itself. In the adolescent the unpredictability of the growth dynamics of the patient greatly diminishes the predictive value of videocephalometric projection [50]. But without doubt, it increases patient involvement and responsibility in decisions. It also results in increased preoperative anxiety but more postoperative satisfaction [41].

Case Illustration

Video cephalometric treatment planning allows quantification of a treatment plan to "retroengineer the numbers to a final plan." In this case, the patient has a Class III open bite with a severe mandibular left laterognathia. The profile is fairly straight, tending more toward convexity than the concavity that would be expected in a Class III pattern. On smile, only 50% of her upper incisor is revealed. A Le Fort I osteotomy with a downgraft of the anterior portion of the maxilla was considered to improve the smile line while closing the bite. Transverse leveling of the maxilla is also required because of the maxillary compensation for the mandibular asymmetry. The Class III discrepancy would have to be treated by either maxillary advancement or mandibular reduction, which raises several questions:

1. Anterior downgraft: How much is required? This is a clinical decision based on the percentage of incisor show on smile and the length of the upper incisor crowns. This must be a clinical judgement rather than a cephalometric assessment because the anterior esthetic relationship will be determined entirely by the patients clinical presentation and not by any cephalometric criteria.
2. Does the maxilla need to come forward or the mandible go back to correct the Class III relationship? Would these movements make the profile unfavorably convex?
3. If the profile does become convex (as would be expected), will genioplasty be required to balance the profile? If a genioplasty is desired, how much is needed to attain the desired end result?

Cephalometric analysis simply cannot answer these questions. In addition, improvisation in the operating room is not very safe either. Mock surgical treatment through video cephalometric planning is an excellent method of testing all these options for facial outcome, virtually arriving at the diagnosis through the testing of the treatment plans. Correction of the malocclusion with facial balance is designed, movement on the computer screen is quantified through the software package, and rather than arriving at a treatment plan that is based on normative values and directing treatment toward that norm, we are outlining the desired profile result on our computer screen. This allowsthe planners to retroengineer the numbers, which enables the surgeon to enter the operating room with a quantitative plan, which in turn maximizes the chances of the planning team to achieve the outcome designed on the computer screen. (Figures 78 – 83)

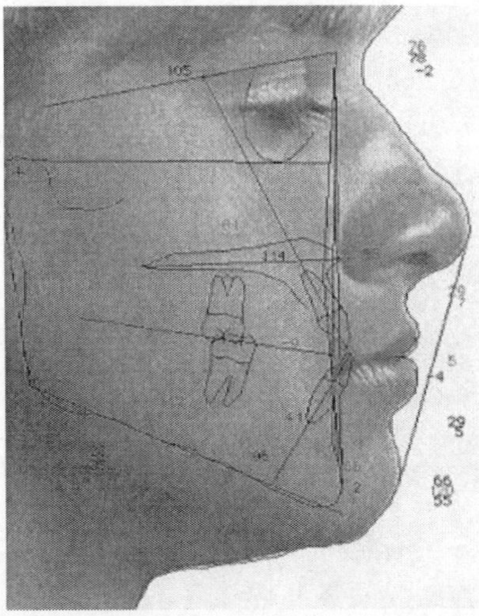

Figure 78. Integrated video cephalogram allows visualization and analysis of hard and soft tissue relationships. Algorithmic prediction is used for profile prediction.

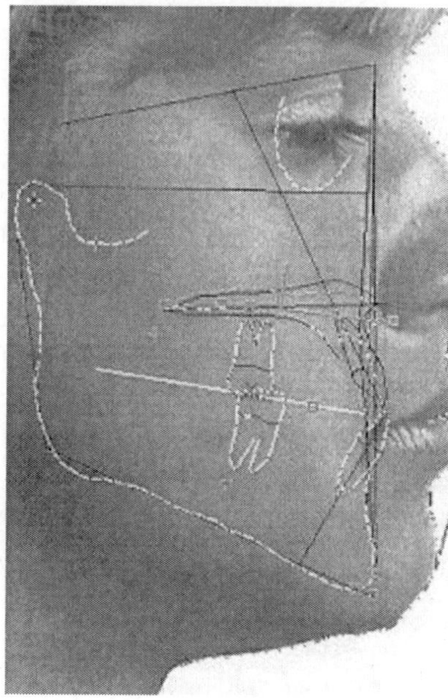

Figure 79. Anterior downgraft of maxilla during LeFort I osteotomy is simulated on cephalometric prediction with "click and drag" function.

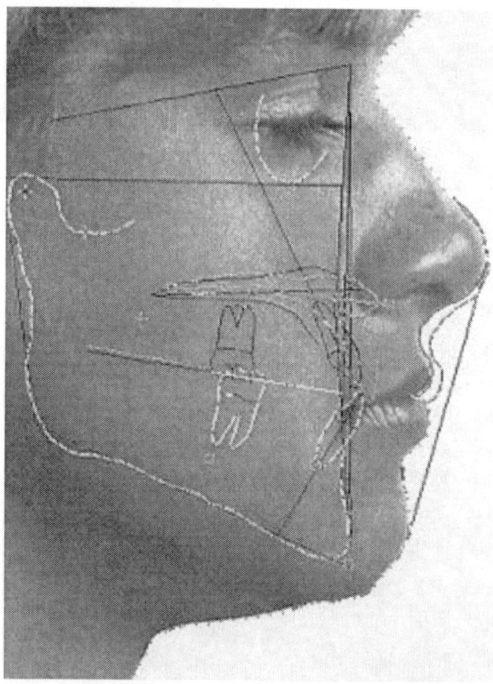

Figure 80. Maxillary advancement and cephalometric prediction improves negative overjet.

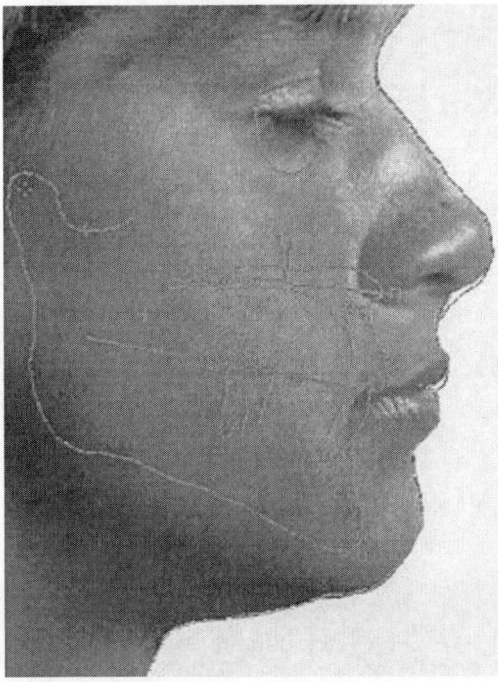

Figure 81. Morphing profile to simulate maxillary advancement demonstrates increase in profile convexity.

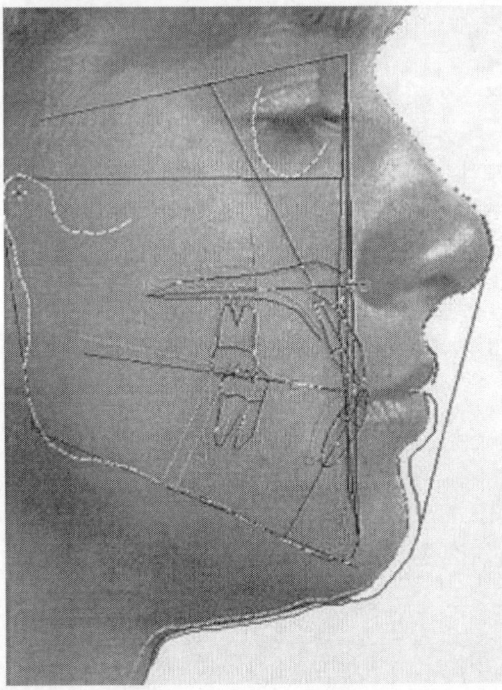

Figure 82. Mandibular reduction also increases profile convexity.

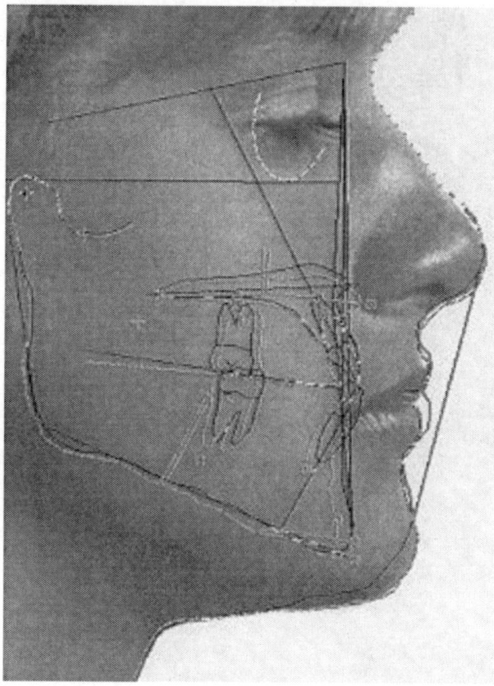

Figure 83. With maxillary and mandibular osteotomies, 4 mm chin advancement results in restoration of profile esthetics. Rhinoplasty is also simulated to refine nasal dorsum and tip.

2. Making the Basic Orthodontic Decisions

Once the basic surgical procedure(s) has been decided upon, the basic orthodontic decisions must be made [24]. These decisions are predicted on the surgical procedure to be done and hence cannot be made before deciding on the surgical procedure(s). The orthodontic decisions that must be made are:

1. What tooth movement is indicated?
2. What are the anchorage requirements for this movement?
3. Do teeth need to be extracted and if required which one?
4. Are there any tooth mass problems?

The first four questions are answered by doing an orthodontic surgical prediction tracing and carefully studying both prediction tracing and the occlusion. The tooth mass problem is best answered by doing an orthodontic setup of the teeth [24].

Necessary Tooth Movement

Once a cephalometric tracing has been done, the tooth movement in both anteroposterior and vertical planes can be easily visualized. Which of the changes will be produced at surgery and which are produced by orthodontics alone must be understood. For instance, if both the vertical and anteroposterior changes in the maxilla that are shown in a prediction tracing for correction of vertical maxillary excess will be accomplished by surgery then there are no orthodontic considerations in the maxilla other than aligning the teeth within the alveolar bone. In some instances the tooth movements called for by a particular cephalometric prediction tracing cannot be accomplished or would require such extreme orthodontic treatment as to be considered unacceptable. In this case the prediction tracing must be redone, usually with an adjunctive procedure to produce a similar result without requiring impossible orthodontic treatment.

Anchorage Requirements

The same cephalometric superimpositions discussed previously are used to determine the anchorage requirements. The changes in the molar and incisor position are studied. For any anchorage requirement in between minimum, moderate maximum conditions the orthodontist will be aware of the anchorage requirements by using the prediction tracing and thus can choose an appropriate sequence of mechanics to produce the desired result.

Teeth to be Extracted and Which One

The need to extract teeth is determined by careful study of both the models and prediction tracings. However, in some cases the surgical procedure can be altered slightly, usually by adding an augmentation genioplasty or by increasing the magnitude of the genioplasty, and by doing so, the need for extractions will no longer be present. Furthermore, it must be appreciated that the lower incisor position is not an absolute; normal position relative to the A-Po line lies within the range of -1mm TO +3mm. When extraction can be avoided by placing the lower incisor at +2 mm or +3 mm, this is generally preferred rather than extracting healthy teeth as long as doing so will not produce an adverse effect on the periodontium.

To this point only the need for extractions in the lower arch is considered, and extractions in the upper arch are been predicted on the need for extraction in the lower. It is not infrequent that a patient with Class II deformity will have crowding in the lower arch, thus requiring extraction, but have a relatively good upper arch, which by itself could be treated without extraction. When this situation exists, the prediction tracing will show the need to move the upper molar forward anywhere from 5-7 mm. Here the clinician has a choice of extracting and moving the molars forward or producing a Class III posterior occlusion. This choice must be left to the orthodontist who will be treating the case. While studies have shown that there is little difference in the number of posterior occlusal contacts between Class I and III posterior occlusion, it is difficult to produce a "good" class III posterior occlusion, and therefore it is often preferable to extract upper second premolars and advance the upper molars to achieve a Class I molar and canine occlusion.

One instance, in which extractions are almost always necessary, even in the absence of crowding, is in the patient who has *no* facial or skeletal asymmetry yet has either a unilateral Class II or Class III malocclusion. When such dental asymmetry exists in the absence of facial asymmetry, the upper, lower, or both dental midlines will usually not be coincident with the facial midline. Rarely, a more subtle situation will be seen when the midlines are well aligned, but the actual arch shape is so asymmetric that the canine and all teeth distal to it on one side are more posteriorly placed in the patient's face than the corresponding teeth on the opposite side of the arch. In either instance asymmetric or unilateral extractions will usually be necessary to produce a satisfactory correction.

One final instance that may require the extraction of teeth is the presence of a severe anterior tooth mass discrepancy. Most frequently, this will require the removal of one lower incisor in patients with very small upper lateral incisors to allow a good posterior occlusion with adequate overbite and overjet and no spacing or restorations in the upper arch.

The decision regarding which teeth to extract can usually be best made from careful study of the cephalometric prediction tracing. Once the tooth movement desired can be visualized as a result of the cephalometric prediction tracing, it is a simple matter to decide if this movement is easier with extraction of the first or the second premolars. When the anterior teeth need to be retracted, the first premolars are the extractions of choice. On the other hand, if the molar teeth are to be advanced, the second premolars become the extractions of choice. Frequently extraction of the first premolars in one arch and the second premolars in the other is done. Importantly in making this decision the orthodontist must remember that the goal is *not* to correct the malocclusion, but to eliminate the dental compensations that are present and preclude effective surgical correction of both the existing malocclusion and facial esthetics.

Certainly other factors such as tooth size and general dental health have a bearing on the specific extractions chosen. Malformed or periodontally involved teeth may need to be extracted to achieve the best overall result, even when doing so will make the orthodontic treatment more difficult or require some modifications of the surgery.

Resolving Tooth Mass Problems

The presence of tooth mass problems has been known to orthodontists for many years, yet these problems seem to be more common in patients with dentofacial deformities. Tooth mass discrepancies are most commonly found in patients with vertical maxillary excess, especially when accompanied by open bite, and in those with mandibular prognathism, although these discrepancies may exist in any patient.

Anterior tooth mass discrepancies of up to 4 mm can usually be corrected by interproximal stripping (recontouring) of the five interproximal areas from canine to canine. If the discrepancy is greater than 4 mm, the removal of a lower incisor will probably be necessary with some recontouring of the upper incisors unless the width of the lower incisor is equal to the discrepancy.

Sequence of Orthodontics and Surgery

It is preferable to perform the orthognathic surgery as early in the patient's treatment as possible for the following reasons: (1) orthodontic precision is greater than surgical precision; thus even when the arches are "perfect" before surgery, a reasonable period of postsurgical orthodontics is invariably necessary. (2) Orthodontic tooth movement is much more rapid following surgery because skeletal and soft tissue relations are normalized and because the rate of bone remodeling is increased as the result of surgery, and (3) the patient's facial appearance is improved earlier in treatment, thus improving both self-image and patient cooperation. To deliberately determine the sequence of orthodontics and surgery, the "two-patient" concept was developed [24].

The Two-Patient Concept

The decision regarding the sequence of orthodontics and surgery is most simply made by using the two-patient concept. This involves (!) making a cephalometric prediction tracing illustrating the effect of surgery when no orthodontic tooth movement is done and (2) doing feasibility model surgery consistent with the planned surgical procedure in which the best possible occlusion before any orthodontic treatment is achieved [24].

Once the feasibility model surgery and prediction tracing are done, these records can be viewed as a second patient, that is, one who manifests the results of the indicated orthognathic surgery prior to any active orthodontic treatment. The orthodontist can then decide if it would be easier to treat the patient after the surgery or if it would be preferable to resolve specific orthodontic problems before surgery.

When this method is used, it becomes obvious that many patients can benefit from having surgery immediately after placing the orthodontic appliances. These are usually patients with vertical maxillary excess for whom the surgeon can produce a Class I malocclusion that is easily treated to completion by routine orthodontic procedures. More frequently, however, because of problems with tooth alignment, leveling, or dental compensations, it is obvious that surgery is best deferred until some orthodontic treatment is completed. *Nevertheless, in all instances feasibility model surgery is beneficial in helping the orthodontist visualize those tooth movements necessary to allow the surgery to be done.* (Figure 84)

Thus the orthodontist can more deliberately direct presurgical efforts toward doing necessary movements, rather than wasting time and effort on nonessential corrections. The decision to do presurgical orthodontic treatment is therefore made on a case-by-case basis. *When presurgical orthodontic treatment is necessary, specific goals for this treatment are established.* Once these goals have been met, surgery can be done and the postsurgical orthodontics readily complete the treatment.

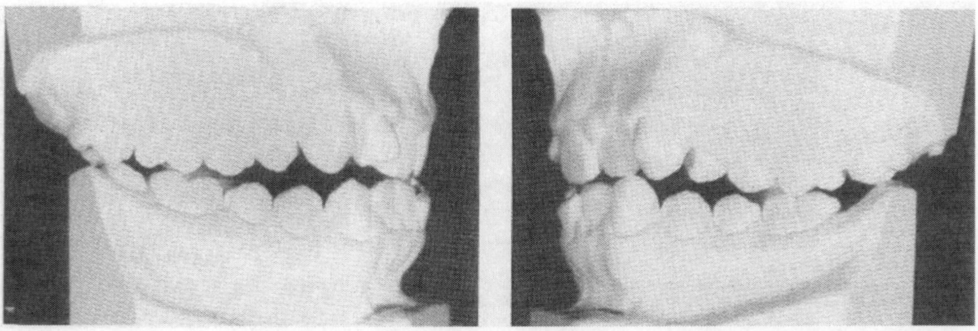

Figure 84. Model Surgery: Right and Left Lateral Views.

Feasibility Model Surgery

The basic reason to perform feasibility model surgery is to determine if the indicated surgical procedure(s) will produce an occlusion that can simply and safely be perfected by subsequent orthodontic treatment [24]. If such an occlusion cannot be produced, the orthodontist can study the model surgery to determine exactly what must be done orthodontically before surgery. This permits the orthodontist to direct his attention toward achieving specific tooth movements. As such, feasibility model surgery is not only done before developing a definitive treatment plan, but it is also routinely done at that time during the presurgical orthodontic treatment when the orthodontist believes the presurgical orthodontic goals have been achieved.

There are basically two types of feasibility model surgery: whole-arch model surgery and segmental model surgery. Whole-arch feasibility model surgery can be done by hand - the dental models are articulated into the best possible occlusion or by doing the same on any simple articulator. Segmental feasibility model surgery is likewise done to determine the best possible occlusion that can be produced. However, it is important in performing segmental feasibility model surgery that it is done on the models in a realistic manner that can be duplicated at surgery. In this regard feasibility model surgery, especially segmental, must be done so that it is both feasible for the surgeon to reproduce it at surgery and feasible for the orthodontist to finish the case from the occlusal result achieved.

Steps in performing segmental feasibility model surgery are:

1. Models are duplicated, trimmed to simulate the anatomy, and mounted on an articulator; a wax bite is used to assure proper occlusion. The roots of the teeth adjacent to where interdental osteotomies or ostectomies will be made are drawn on the cast as they exist in the radiographs. A referent line is marked on the models about 5 above the tooth root apices. (Figure 85)
2. The teeth and alveolus are sectioned from the upper model along the reference line made approximately 5 mm above the tooth root apices. (Figure 86)

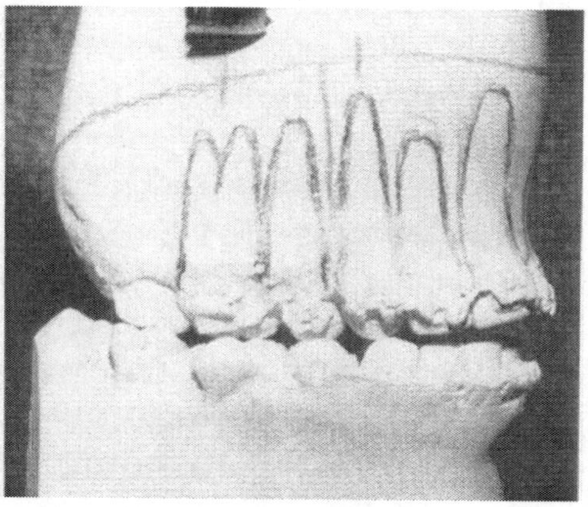

Figure 85. Model with roots of teeth and referent lines marked.

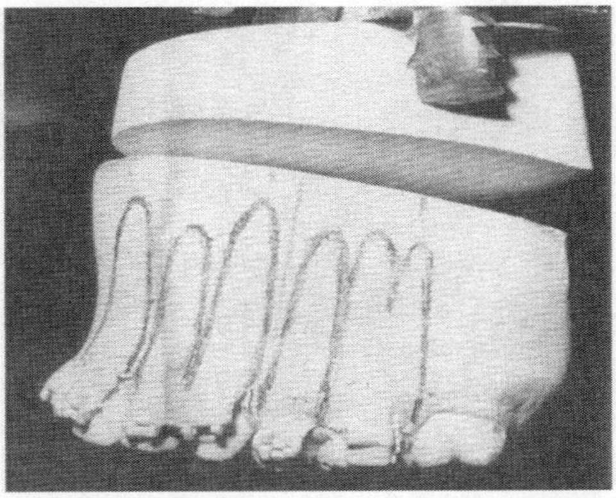

Figure 86. Sectioned teeth and alveolus in upper model.

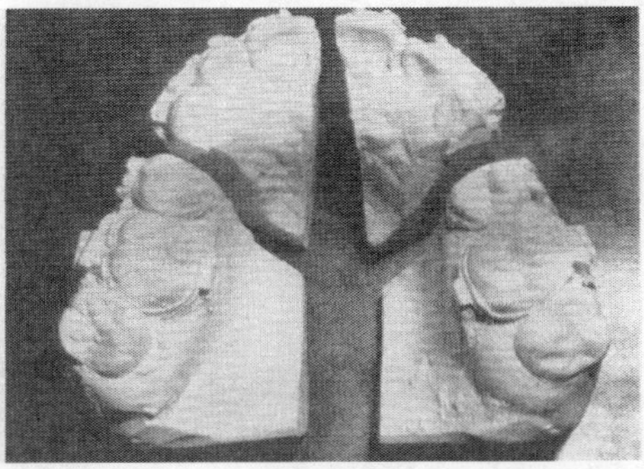

Figure 87. Sectioned upper model.

3. The maxilla is sectioned into the appropriate segments, taking care not to involve the tooth roots. (Figure 87)
4. The anterior segment or segments are placed into their best occlusal relationship with the lower teeth and held into this position with soft wax. Every effort is made to establish a Class I canine occlusion with normal overbite and overjet. (Figure 88)

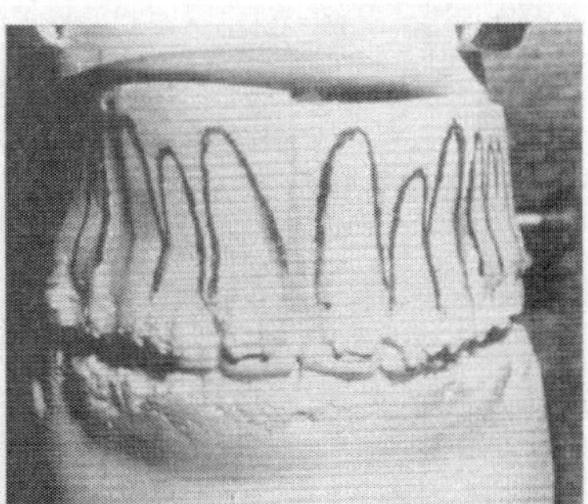

Figure 88. Proper anterior occlusion on cast.

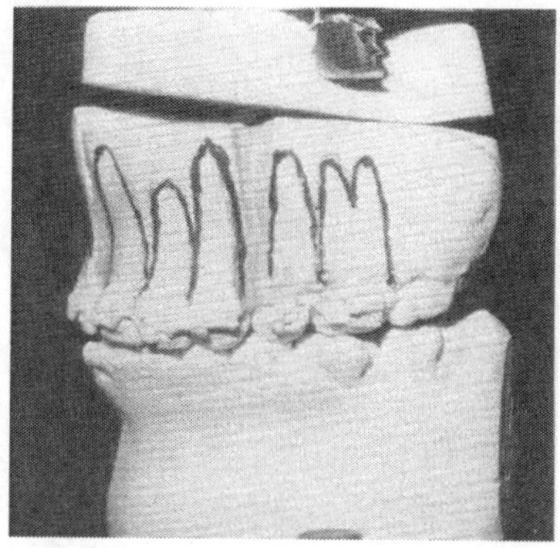

Figure 89. Proper posterior occlusion on cast.

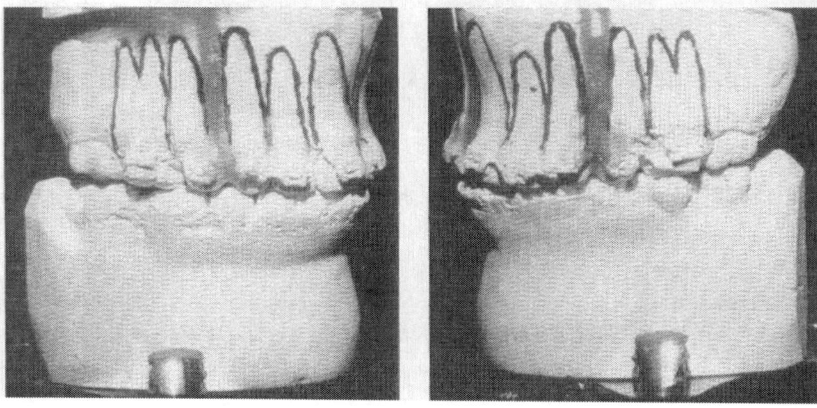

Figure 90. Joining of segments with sticky wax.

5. Each posterior segment is subsequently placed into its best occlusal relationship and held into position with soft wax. The soft wax permits the segments to be simply adjusted during their initial set-up. (Figure 89)
6. Once the best possible occlusion is achieved, the segments are joined to one another and to the base with a heavy application of sticky wax to prevent them from moving. (Figure 90)

When a lower subapical procedure is planned in conjunction with other maxillary or mandibular surgery, the lower subapical osteotomy is almost always completed first. The objective is to produce as ideal a lower arch as possible; thus the lower curve of Spee must be as flat as possible, the midline maintained or corrected to the facial midline, and any spaces where interdental osteotomies have been must be as small as possible, consistent with good surgical technique.

1. The models are trimmed to simulate the anatomy and mounted on an articulator; a wax bite is used to assure proper occlusion. The roots of the teeth adjacent to where interdental osteotomies or osteotomies will be made are drawn on the casts. (Figure 91)

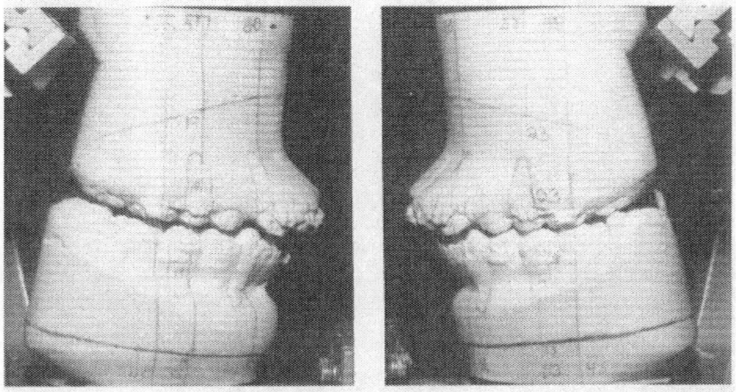

Figure 91. Models with osteotomy drawings.

2. The illustrated case is to be done for correction of bimaxillary protrusion and thus the entire lower dentoalveolar segment is sectioned from the lower cast at a safe level below the tooth root apices. Appropriate plaster is removed from both the interdental sites and cast base to allow repositioning of the lower segment into its desired position; care is taken not to involve the tooth roots. (Figure 92)
3. The anterior mandibular subapical segment is positioned to achieve the best possible arch form and curve of Spee and held with soft wax. (Figure 93)
4. After the lower subapical osteotomy is completed, the upper arch is done as discussed earlier. (Figure 94)

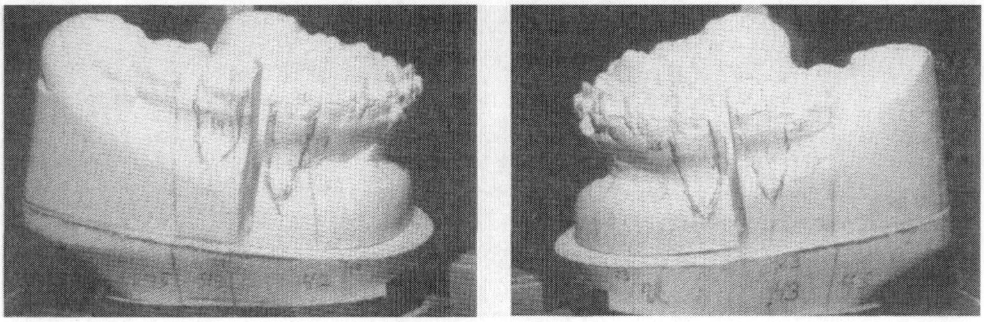

Figure 92. Repositioning of the lower segment.

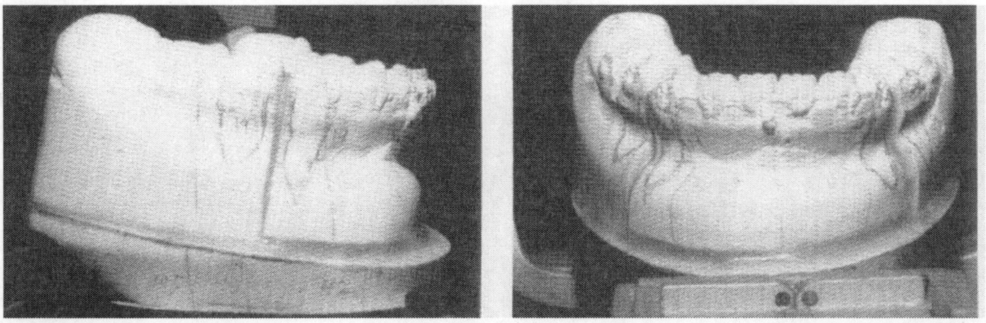

Figure 93. Repositioning of the anterior segment.

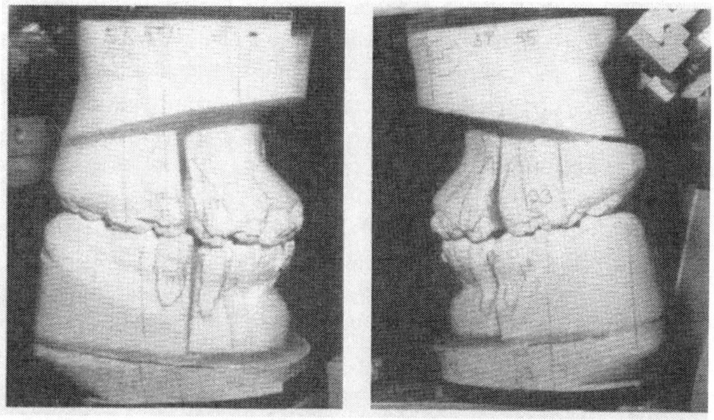

Figure 94. Completed Setup.

Once the feasibility model surgery is done, it is evaluated by the orthodontist who will be responsible for finishing the case from the occlusion that can be produced at surgery. The orthodontist is responsible for the decision to proceed with the orthognathic surgery or to delay the same. If the occlusion produced by the feasibility model surgery produces a situation that is difficult to correct orthodontically, then surgery is delayed until the orthodontist moves the teeth into a position in which those specific problems are not encountered. As orthodontic treatment is progressing and the orthodontist believes he has achieved his presurgical goals, new models are made, the feasibility model surgery is redone, and the results are again examined. Once the occlusion that can be produced by surgery is acceptable to the orthodontist, the patient is ready for surgery [24].

Chapter 8

PRE-SURGICAL ORTHODONTICS

The orthodontic treatment to bring teeth in correct position usually involves removing dental compensation, which means that the dental relationships temporarily become worse and therefore presurgical orthodontics is usually called as ***reverse orthodontics*** [1]. With the "decompensation" of the dentition and the apparent "worsening of the malocclusion," the stage is set for the surgical phase of treatment. The surgeon is thus presented with a case in which the problem is fully exposed, all of the malocclusion's skeletal features are clearly identifiable, and an optimal surgical correction is possible. By decompensating the dentition and making things look worse before they get better, the orthodontist is allowing the surgeon to move the jaws the maximum amount that he may require to provide a correct skeletal relationship with fewer limitations being presented by inappropriate tooth positioning.

The orthodontic treatment objectives for an orthognathic case are, in the vast majority of cases, entirely opposite those that might be employed if the case were to be treated by conventional orthodontic methods alone. In addition, it is often found that the extraction pattern demanded in an orthognathic case is the reverse of that seen in a comparable orthodontic case. For instance, the classic pattern of extracting upper first premolars and lower second premolars in a conventional Class II case might be replaced by a pattern that entailed extraction of upper second premolars and lower first premolars if the case were to be treated orthognathically. The objective of this extraction pattern is to establish a full-step Class II molar and canine relationship where this is not already present, thus allowing the maximum possible surgical correction of the underlying skeletal deformity [51].

Goals of presurgical orthodontics:

1. ***Positioning the teeth over basal bone***
2. ***Aligning and leveling the teeth***
3. ***Adjusting for tooth size discrepancy***
4. ***Correction of rotated teeth***
5. ***Coordinating upper and lower arches*** *[1]*

PRESURGICAL OBJECTIVES

1. Intra-Arch Objectives

In the initial stages of treatment, orthognathic and conventional orthodontic mechanics have some similar objectives like correction of arch length deficiencies, elimination of rotations, and overall arch-alignment are all common features. Tooth-size discrepancies must be identified and eliminated preoperatively to permit achievement of the best possible anterior occlusal interdigitation at surgery. Procedures such as interdental enamel reduction, extraction of a mandibular incisor where indicated, and the distribution of excess space due to diminutive lateral incisors must be concluded prior to surgery. Intra-arch mechanics in orthognathic cases should be designed to achieve the ultimately desired postsurgical interdigitation and allow for the establishment of Class I canine and molar relationships after surgical treatment. Achievement of these objectives will require that the maxillary and mandibular teeth be positioned in as "ideal" relationships to their underlying osseous bases as possible. If extractions are necessary to accomplish the desired objectives, then the extraction sites should be closed unless segmentalized surgical closure is planned. In orthognathic cases it is necessary to establish the correct incisor and molar torque prior to surgery as mechanics aimed at achieving these ends, if delayed until after the surgery, may tend to cause relapse, such as the return of open bites [51].

2. Anteroposterior (Sagittal) Objectives

In most malocclusions in which there is a severe underlying skeletal deformity, the dentition has often maintained some occlusal contact and interdigitation by the teeth compensating in their positions for the skeletal problem. These dental compensations are manifested in all three planes of space but are most apparent in the sagittal dimension. In skeletal Class II cases, commonly seen dental compensations include very protrusive mandibular incisors and upright maxillary incisors [51]. (Figure 95)

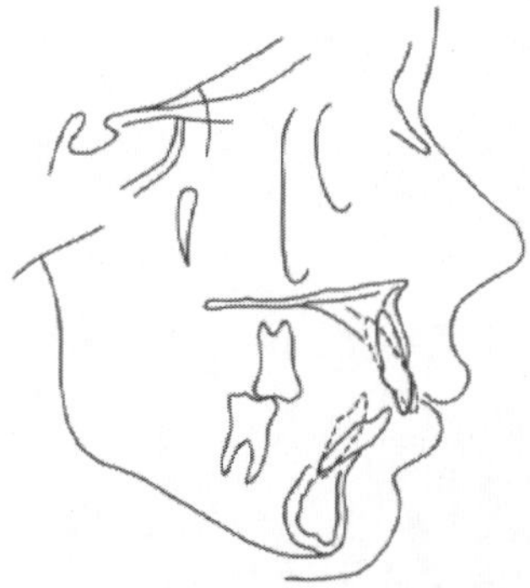

Figure 95. Class II case demonstrating incisor positions before (—) and after (----) dental decompensation.

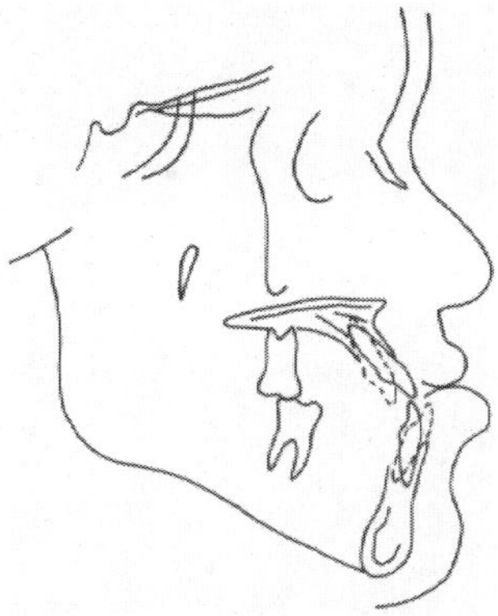

Figure 96. Class III case demonstrating incisor positions before (—) and after (----) dental decompensation.

Conversely, in skeletal Class III cases, the mandibular incisors are often found to be retroclined while the maxillary incisors are commonly flared forward. (Figure 96)

Since the presurgical objectives in orthognathic cases include positioning the incisors in axial relationships that are as "ideal" as possible, it will often be necessary to "decompensate" the incisors with orthodontic mechanotherapy. Achievement of this "decompensation" objective will often necessitate the use of Class III elastics in Class II patients to upright the mandibular incisors and reciprocally advance the maxillary molars. Conversely, Class II elastics might be used in Class III patients to retract the maxillary incisors and to bring the mandibular molars forward. (Figure 97)

Similar principles apply to anchorage requirements in Class II orthognathic cases the greatest anchorage requirement is in the mandibular arch for retraction of the usually proclined incisors.

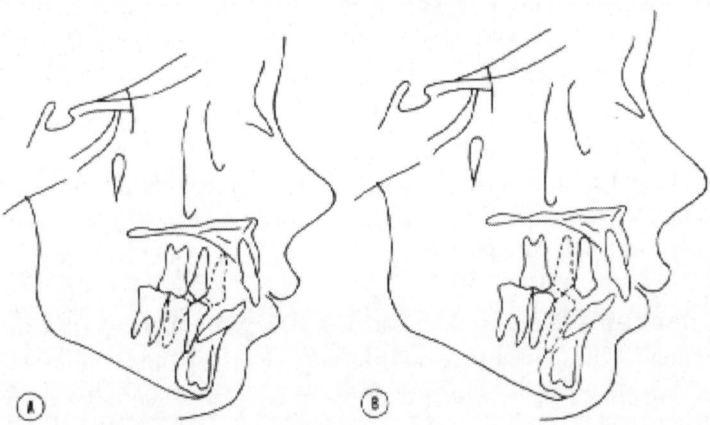

Figure 97. A, Class ll case with upper first and lower second premolar extraction requiring maximum anchorage in the maxillary arch using conventional orthodontic techniques to retract the incisors. B, Class II case with upper second and lower first premolar extraction requiring maximum mandibular arch anchorage to retract the proclined incisors prior to orthognathic surgery.

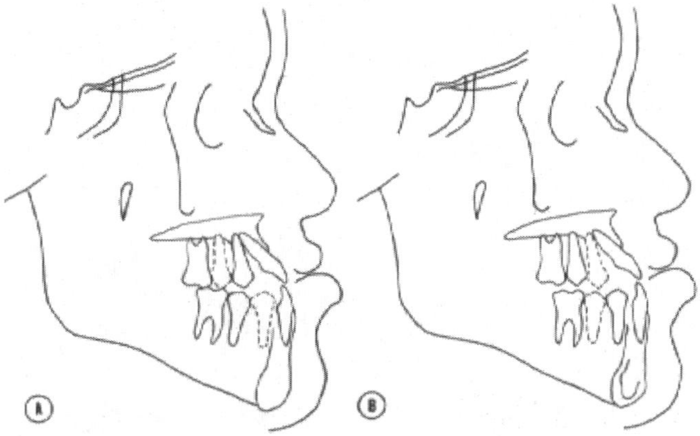

Figure 98. A, Class lll case with extraction of upper second and lower first premolars requiring maximum anchorage in the mandibular arch to retract the incisors by conventional orthodontic techniques. B, Class III case with extraction of upper first and lower second premolars requiring maximum anchorage in the maxilla to retract the incisors prior to orthognathic surgery.

Conversely, Class III cases often require maximum anchorage in the maxilla and minimal anchorage in the mandible in association with a pattern of extraction of maxillary first premolars and mandibular second premolars where this is indicated to alleviate the dental compensations and produce a full-step Class III molar relationship prior to surgical intervention. (Figure 98)

3. Transverse Objectives

When considering the need for orthognathic mechanics to correct problems in the transverse dimension, it is essential to determine whether the problem manifested is skeletal or dental in nature. When it has been determined whether the problems identified are skeletal or dental in nature and whether they involve absolute or relative discrepancies, the optimum course of treatment becomes obvious. Skeletal discrepancies should not be masked by compensatory dental movements. Such procedures as expansion through headgear, arch wire, or elastic therapy are not recommended; nor are attempts at arch coordination by means of continuous arch wires recommended since these procedures have a high relapse potential. Compensations such as tipped molars and premolars should be corrected, and the correct buccal segment torque should be established prior to surgical intervention. Failure to achieve these goals may result in the surgical expansion being found inadequate, as postsurgical orthodontic correction of these problems will usually involve some lingual movement of the maxillary buccal cusps. In cases in which there is an isolated skeletal transverse discrepancy and no other maxillary surgery is anticipated, a lateral maxillary osteotomy (corticotomy) followed by rapid palatal expansion may be the procedure of choice. Where a skeletal maxillary discrepancy is combined with other maxillary problems, multiple-segment maxillary surgical procedures are indicated. To avoid "building in" adverse dental relapse potential, the application of segmental arch orthodontic mechanics is advisable prior to segmental maxillary surgery. The individual arch-wire segments should correspond to the anticipated surgical segments as determined by the patient's malocclusion and arch form.

Cases with minor dental transverse discrepancies are suitable for routine continuous arch therapy, including full-arch coordination prior to surgery [51].

4. Vertical Objectives

The two principal objectives of orthognathic mechanics in the vertical plane prior to surgery are the avoidance of adverse dental relapse potential and the maximizing of the speed and efficiency of treatment. In cases in which anterior facial height is to be reduced surgically (open bites or open bite tendencies) the major portion of orthodontic tooth movement should be accomplished prior to surgery. When the open bite has resulted in only minimal to moderate curves in either arch, the use of a continuous arch wire and presurgical leveling is indicated. This is also true where extractions are required or where excessive anterior spacing exists. Where anchorage requirements dictate the use of a headgear, care should be taken when a high-pull headgear is used, as any resultant intrusion of the maxillary molars may tend to rebound after surgery. Any postsurgical extrusion of the maxillary molars may lead to the return of an open bite. Avoidance of intrusive mechanics in the posterior region and concurrent avoidance of any extrusive mechanics in the anterior region will also facilitate maximum surgical correction of the deformity. To avoid excessive extrusion or intrusion of teeth and potential adverse relapse tendencies, careful consideration should be given to surgical rather than orthodontic correction of severely accentuated or reversed curves of Spee. Segmental orthodontic therapy should be carried out where necessary, possibly in both the maxilla and the mandible, prior to corresponding segmental surgery, with the osteotomy sites being where the "break" in the occlusal plane occurs.

In those patients who exhibit a deep bite tendency and short anterior face height, the major portion of the orthodontic mechanics, especially relative to the leveling of the mandibular occlusal plane, should be postponed until after the surgery. To obtain the optimum in efficiency of treatment, stability, and esthetic change, the leveling of an accentuated mandibular curve of Spee should be postponed until after the surgical procedure, while the maxillary arch can usually be leveled easily prior to the surgery. In this way the difficult leveling process in the mandible may be easily accomplished mechanically after surgery by means of vertical elastics, since the postsurgical occlusion will be primarily on the molars and incisors. Presurgical leveling would have to overcome the heavy bite forces often associated with deep bites. (Figure 99)

This treatment sequence tends to enhance the stability of mandibular advancement procedures, since the presence of a deep bite presurgically will facilitate the introduction of an opening component of rotation of the mandible during the advancement. This opening rotation tends to be more stable than straight forward or closing rotations, which include an increase in posterior face height. The presence of a deep bite prior to surgery will also facilitate the maximum esthetic improvement in the patient's short facial height, since the downward and forward mandibular movement will augment the increase in anterior facial height [51].

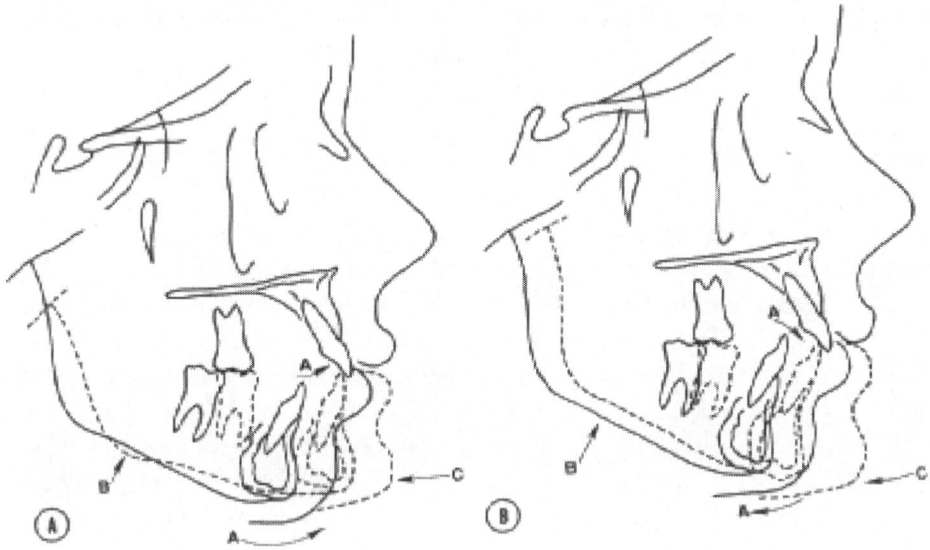

Figure 99. A, Class II case leveled presurgically (—). Surgical changes (----) noted include: A, Closing mandibular rotation; B, increased posterior face height; C, no increase in anterior face height. B, The same Class II case not leveled presurgically (—). Surgical changes (----) noted include: A, Opening mandibular rotation; B, no increase in posterior face height; C, increased anterior face height.

Procedures that need to be done before surgery include –

- Alignment: primarily by tipping, flexible round wire (16 mil austenitic NiTi best)
- Intrusion (leveling): segmented arch technique required, stabilizing lingual arches needed.
- Arch compatibility: to be careful regarding second molars' vertical position and canine widths [2].

Procedures that can be done before and/or after surgery –

- Post. crossbite correction: no orthodontic expansion before surgery in a patient who will have surgical expansion; can leave up to half cusp crossbite for correction after surgery.
- Leveling by extrusion: easier and more efficient after surgery; partial leveling with continuous arch wires can be done before surgery [2].

Procedures necessary after surgery –

- Extrusion (Settling and leveling).
- Root paralleling at osteotomy sites.
- Detailed tooth positioning: all these to be completed in 4-6 months [2].

SELECTION OF THE APPLIANCE

Orthodontic appliance for surgical orthodontic patients is used not only to move teeth but also to stabilize them against the stresses encountered at surgery and during maxillomandibular fixation. Two major fixed appliance systems are in use at present:

1. The Edgewise appliance with its myriad of modifications.
2. The Begg's appliance [2].

The difficulty of doing this with Begg's appliance is a strong argument against its use in surgical patients. It is not impossible to do good surgical orthodontic treatment using Begg's appliance but it is significantly more difficult and problematic. Therefore straight wire appliance is recommended for use with surgical patients. Other considerations in choosing appliance for surgical patients include [2]:

Esthetics

The most esthetic appliances today are the lingual appliances. But these are not recommended for surgical patients due to the following reasons –

- Impossible to use the appliance for stabilizing the teeth during surgery or IMF. If a lingual appliance is being used, it will be necessary to place labial appliance as well, at least temporarily, for use in the operating room and in the immediate post surgical rehabilitation period.
- Post operative patients have difficulty in mouth opening for the first few months when the postsurgical orthodontics must be done. This greatly complicates the already difficult process of using a lingual appliance.

Tooth colored brackets (plastic and ceramic) can also be used to enhance esthetics but their use is not recommended in an orthognathic patient as –

Plastic brackets – Not suited for surgery as they tend to fracture, and bracket slot is not good enough to provide good torque control.

Ceramic brackets are stronger than plastic brackets, and provide good torque control. But they are brittle and can fracture so impacts should be avoided during treatment, especially during surgery. They are satisfactory for surgical treatment, but should be limited to the upper anteriors only, and the surgeon must be prepared to use alternative stabilizing methods (like arch bars) if the brackets fracture in the OT [2].

Slot Size

Either slot size – 18 or 22 – is good enough for surgery, as long as a full sized wire is placed in the slot. But when segmented arch mechanics needs to be employed, 22 slot is preferable, as the individual segments can be well stabilized with 21x25 ss wires [2].

Bonding Vs. Banding

It is usually advisable to bond anteriors and band posteriors. When there are periodontal problems, bands are to be avoided, due to difficulty in keeping the area clean. A fully bonded appliance is preferred in that circumstance, despite the greater chance of appliance problems [2].

Appliance Modifications

Although Pre Adjusted Edgewise Appliance brackets are recommended for surgery, few things must be kept in mind [2]:

1. All prescriptions cannot be used for surgical patients. Extreme prescriptions must be avoided. "Extraction series" brackets tend to have a high amount of tip on the canine and premolar brackets which result in roots converging into the extraction space. This can cause problems in case of segmental osteotomies. Hence roots should not be converging in the extraction space. On the other hand, the opposite side bracket should not be placed, as it would cause too much root separation, and increase the time required for post- surgical orthodontics.
2. All teeth should be included in the strap-up. Mandibular second molars can be included before surgery, but it is better to include maxillary molars after surgery, as they have a tendency to extrude. This can interfere with surgical positioning of the jaw bases. If the maxillary second molars are included before surgery, they must be kept depressed using a step bend.
3. Auxiliary molar tubes and headgear tubes should be present, and molars should have lingual attachments to aid in use of cross elastics.
4. Brackets with adequate mesio-distal and rotational control (twin brackets or single brackets with rotational wings) to be used.
5. Integral hooks in the brackets- these help in stabilization during surgery and for attaching elastics during post surgical orthodontics. Long hooks should be avoided, as they make oral hygiene maintenance difficult. Some surgeons however feel that the brackets may get dislodged if these hooks are used for stabilization, and prefer to use hooks on the archwire instead.

Steps in Orthodontic Preparation of the Patient [2]

Alignment of the Arch

Alignment is not different for patients who will have surgery. Guiding principle basically is the initial tipping of the teeth into their correct position, using undersized, round and resilient wires. This permits free sliding, freedom to tip mesio-distally and labio-lingually, and light continuous forces, with longer range of action. Bodily movement is not only unnecessary but also undesirable.

Leveling of the Arch

Unlike non-surgical orthodontics, leveling of the arch in all surgical patients is not necessary pre-surgically. Often it is advantageous to leave some amount of vertical discrepancy and allow the arch to be leveled surgically. Also, a large amount of leveling is also done post-surgically. When the mandible is moved forward or back surgically, the final vertical height of the face is determined by the **position of the lower incisors**.

- If it is desired to increase the face height → the lower incisors should not be intruded, and leveling of the arch should be done post-surgically, by extrusion.
- In patients with normal or excessive face height, the lower incisors must be intruded pre-surgically.

If segmental procedures are to be done, the teeth should be leveled within the segments, and the final leveling among the segments will be done post-surgically.

Antero–Posterior Positioning of the Incisors

Just as the position of incisors vertically will determine postsurgical face height because the surgeon must bring the teeth together at the time of operation, so the antero-posterior position of the teeth affect the amount the jaws that can be moved sagittaly at surgery. Except that the goal of the treatment is often is not to reduce but to increase the overjet or reverse overjet before surgery, the orthodontic mechanotherapy needed to establish presurgical incisor position is no different from what is done in routine treatment. The amount of incisor retraction is a function of the anchorage available, which the orthodontist must control. Either sliding mechanics or loop mechanics can be used to vary anteroposterior position of the incisors. Invariably, a slight rebound follows tooth movement and also there is also a period of IMF, which tends to augment the forces of relapse. So modest overtreatment of incisor position is desirable.

Segmental Surgeries

In these cases, the axial inclination of the anterior teeth in the anterior segment must be established pre-surgically. If the axial inclination is corrected surgically, it can cause the canine to be elevated from the occlusal plane, and proper post-surgical poisoning of the canine becomes difficult (Figure 100).

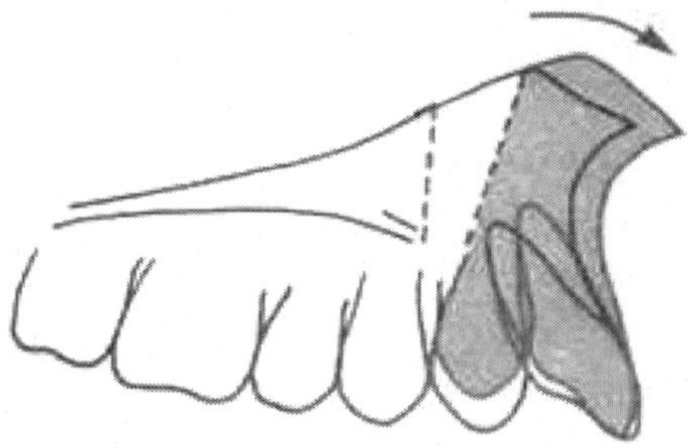

Figure 100. Correction of axial inclination of upper canine.

If the osteotomy site is at an extraction site, up to half the extraction space should be left open so as to allow for the osteotomy cut.

Small amount of space can be left to help in some minor corrections post-surgically.

Arch Compatibility

The final step is to assure that the maxillary and mandibular archforms are compatible to each other, so that the teeth fit into each other after surgery. This includes **shape and width**.

Usually, one of the arches has a U shape and the other has a V shape. The narrower regions need to be expanded. This can be done by using co-ordinated arch wires from the beginning, and slowly proceeding to heavier archwires. Sometimes exaggerated arch wire forms may be needed to correct the archform. After archform correction, the roots will have to be torqued, so as to prevent cuspal interferences. But no more than 2-3 mm per side of dental expansion should be done, anything more than that should be done surgically. All the expansion does not need to be done before surgery. Upto a half cusp cross-bite can be left to be corrected post-surgically, when the occlusal interferences have been relieved. A slight amount of arch incompatibility can be tolerated when splints are used. Confirming the arch compatibility clinically can be difficult. A Class II patient can protrude his mandible, and this can give some idea as to anterior compatibility. But this is not possible in a class III patient. Checking the compatibility of a set of study casts taken just before presurgical preparation can help confirm arch compatibility.

At the end of the pre-surgical phase, the patient should be in a full sized rectangular steel wire which will help stabilize the teeth during surgery.

Presurgical Procedures to Be Carried Out in Different Malocclusions.

Class II

The presurgical orthodontic treatment most often required by the Class II Division I malocclusion is leveling of the curve of Spee, expansion of the maxillary intercanine distance, and the lingual tipping of mandibular incisors. Class II division 2 cases on other hand; usually require labial tipping of the maxillary central incisors and leveling of the curve of Spee [51].

Class III

The presurgical tooth movements that need to be produced in the Class III cases are the expansion of intercanine distance in the maxilla, the labial tipping of lower incisors, and the lingual tipping of upper incisors. Without the uprighting of mandibular incisors presurgically, a certain amount of relapse should be expected [51].

Open-Bite

In open-bite cases, the alveolar processes often are already elongated. Also, during intermaxillary fixation, a certain amount of extrusion of anterior teeth tends to occur. To help in overcorrection of the open bite and to avoid excessive elongation of the alveolus, the anterior teeth should not be extruded presurgically by orthodontic means in an attempt to close the bite. If the upper posterior teeth are over erupted during the growth of the patient, which in many times is the case, an attempt should be made to intrude these teeth prior to surgery [51].

Asymmetry

In cases of asymmetry, as in all malocclusions of skeletal origin, correcting the teeth malpositions themselves on their respective bases is an attempt to achieve occlusion with the opposing arch. The dental compensation of the maxillary teeth is therefore a shift toward the asymmetrical mandible, while the mandibular teeth tend to shift away from the midline of the mandible, toward the maxilla. To correct this lateral shift of the mandible, the teeth should be positioned orthodontically prior to surgical treatment. Each arch should be centered over its respective basal bone, with the maxillary teeth centered with the facial midline and the mandibular teeth with the midline of the chin. This then enables the surgeon to align the midline of the chin with that of the face at the time the malocclusion is corrected [51].

Chapter 9

Definitive Immediate Pre-Surgical Planning

Definitive immediate surgical planning is done after completing the necessary presurgical orthodontic treatment and after determining that the patient is ready for surgery by feasibility model surgery. This planning involves:

1. making a surgical cephalometric prediction tracing,
2. performing definitive model surgery, and
3. constructing a surgical occlusal splint when indicated [24].

Immediately prior to surgery, after all the presurgical orthodontic objectives have been accomplished, the orthodontist should take a complete set of presurgical records. These records should consist of accurate models (for simulating model surgery and for splint fabrication), a centric relation recording, a face-bow transfer and mounting where indicated, a cephalometric head film in centric relation with lips in repose, and facial as well as intraoral photographs.

The face-bow transfer and mounting on an adjustable articulator are advisable in cases exhibiting significant asymmetries as well as in cases requiring maxillary and combined maxillary and mandibular procedures. Only in this way can model surgery adequately simulate the necessary surgical moves and the resulting mandibular anatomic response.

Surgical Cephalometric Prediction Tracing

The surgical cephalometric prediction tracing is made from a cephalometric radiograph obtained shortly before surgery and after the presurgical orthodontic treatment has been completed.

Its purpose is to plan the details of the surgical movement (skeletal): the size and shape of osteotomies, the intraosseous wire positions, the size of bone grafts, the necessity and magnitude of adjunctive procedures such as genioplasty, and optimal soft tissue changes [46].

Unlike the combined orthodontic-surgical prediction tracings, the surgeon is bound by the position of the teeth that has been produced by the presurgical orthodontic treatment. As such, the surgical cephalometric prediction tracings, while similar in technique, are more simply and directly done. These prediction tracings provide much of the essential information required to properly perform the surgery. Furthermore, by superimposing the prediction tracing on the cephalometric radiograph obtained immediately following surgery, the accuracy of the predicted surgical changes can be studied. Significant discrepancies between the predicted and actually obtained result may warrant additional surgical intervention before the patient leaves the hospital.

Mandibular Advancement with Augmentation Genioplasty [46]

All structures are traced from the presurgical cephalometric radiograph and is called the tracing (solid line). (Figure 101)

The prediction (heavy dashed line) is begun by tracing the entire distal mandible, the mandibular teeth, and the soft tissue chin on a new piece of tracing acetate overlaid on the tracing. This approximates the actual anatomy (geometry) of the distal mandible that will be repositioned at surgery. (Figure 102)

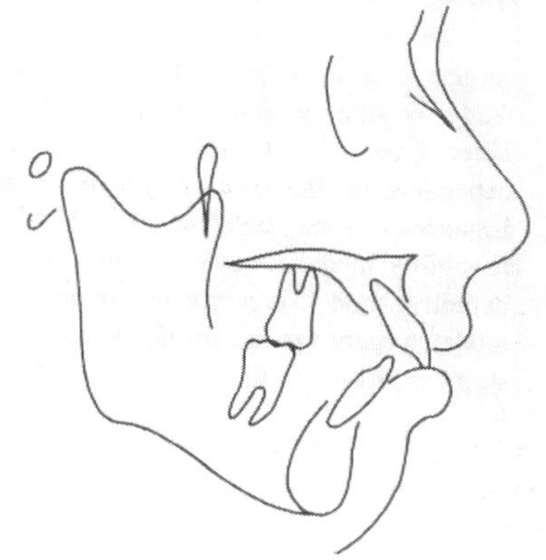

Figure 101. Tracing.

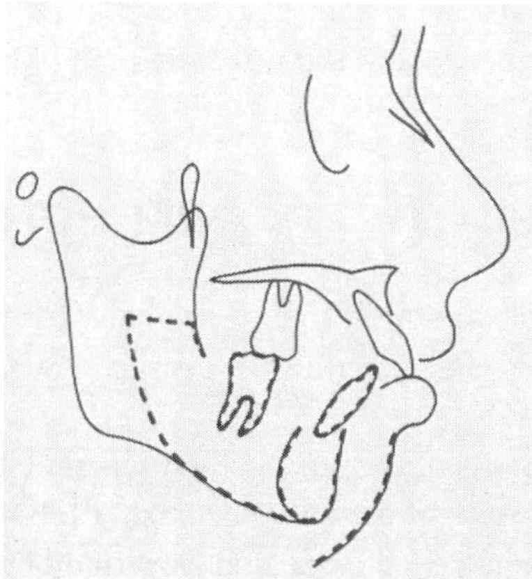

Figure 102. Prediction tracing.

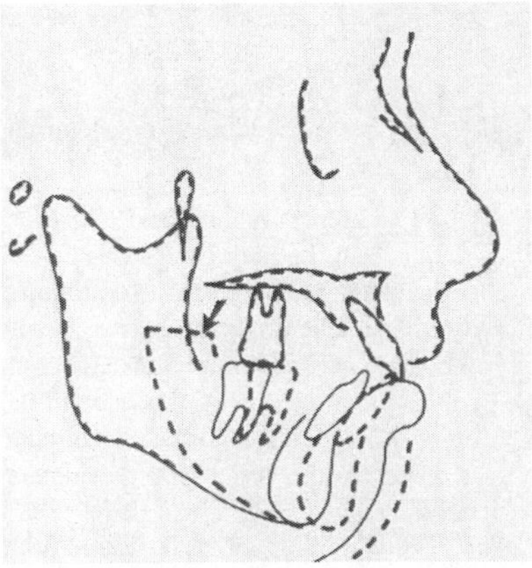

Figure 103. Prediction tracing with mandibular advancement.

The prediction is moved forward on the tracing to produce the ideal occlusal relations, and the stable structures, including the proximal mandible, are traced. The relation of the proximal and distal ramus segments are noted (see arrow) so that the proper relations of the intraosseous holes and wires can be achieved at surgery. This is essential for good stability because proper placement of the intraosseous holes and wires affects control of the proximal segments and condyle positions. (Figure 103)

Frankfort horizontal (FH) and subnasale perpendicular are constructed on the prediction, and the horizontal distance between soft tissue pogonion and subnasale perpendicular is measured to determine the need for, and the magnitude (millimeters) of an augmentation genioplasty. Ideally the soft tissue chin is 4 mm behind the subnasale perpendicular. When an osseous augmentation genioplasty is done, the soft tissue pogonion moves forward 0.7 mm for each 1.0 mm of bony advancement. Accordingly, the specific amount of osseous advancement is determined as it relates to the soft tissue parameters described by the subnasale perpendicular. (Figure 104)

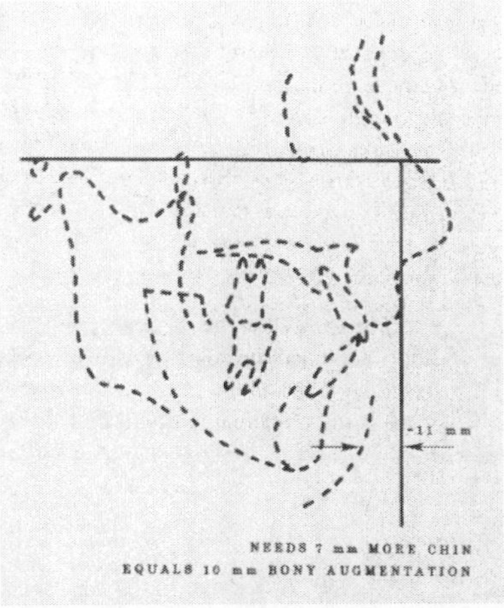

Figure 104. Prediction tracing with FH plane and Sn perpendicular.

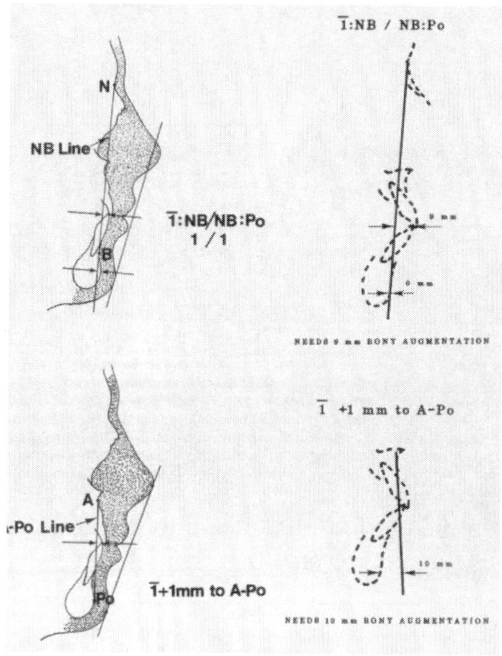

Figure 105. Prediction tracing with NB: Po and A-Po relations.

No single parameter ideally defines the anteroposterior chin relation. Thus the NB: Po and A-Po relations are also studied to determine the ideal position of the chin relative to these hard tissue landmarks. Ideally the incisal edge of the lower incisor lies equally as far ahead of the NB line as does the bony pogonion. Also, the incisal edge of the lower incisor ideally lies 1 mm ± 2 mm ahead of the A-Po line. By adding the information from these two relations to that obtained from the subnasale perpendicular evaluation, the chin can be optimally repositioned. Usually the desired amount of augmentation will be nearly the same; however, a discrepancy may exist when the soft tissue covering the chin is extremely thin or (rarely) when it is excessively thick. (Figure 105)

If considerable variance exists between these parameters, as a general principle the bony chin is not to be advanced anteriorly further than the lower incisor position.

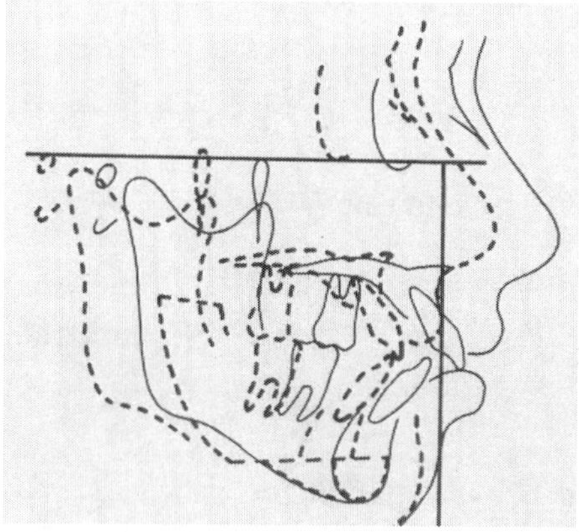

Figure 106. Prediction tracing with genioplasty.

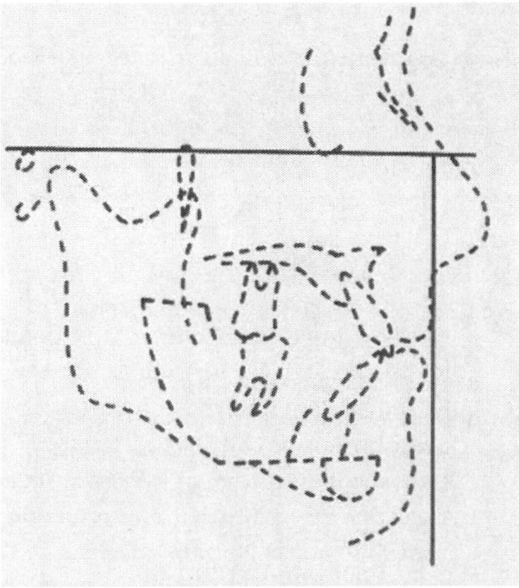

Figure 107. Prediction tracing with completed soft tissues.

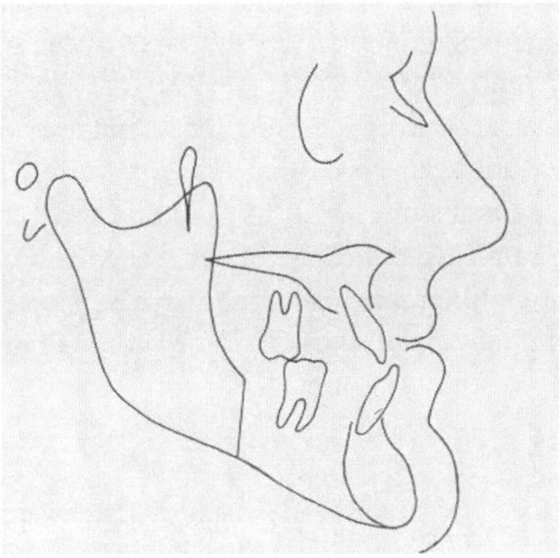

Figure 108. Prediction tracing with sagittal osteotomy line.

After both the inferior mandibular area (chin) where the genioplasty is to be added and the soft tissue chin are erased from the prediction, the proposed genioplasty is added to the prediction by sliding the prediction backward on the tracing until the desired amount of bony augmentation is produced. The bony augmentation is traced, and the corresponding soft tissue change is illustrated, remembering that the soft tissue change is somewhat less than the skeletal augmentation (0.7:1 bony augmentation and 0.9:1 for alloplastic augmentation). (Figure 106)

The prediction is finished by completing the soft tissues of the lower lip. (Figure 107)

Mandibular Setback with Reduction Genioplasty

All structures are traced from the presurgical cephalometric radiograph. A vertical line is placed on the mandible to indicate the approximate position of the vertical component of the sagittal osteotomy. (Figure 108)

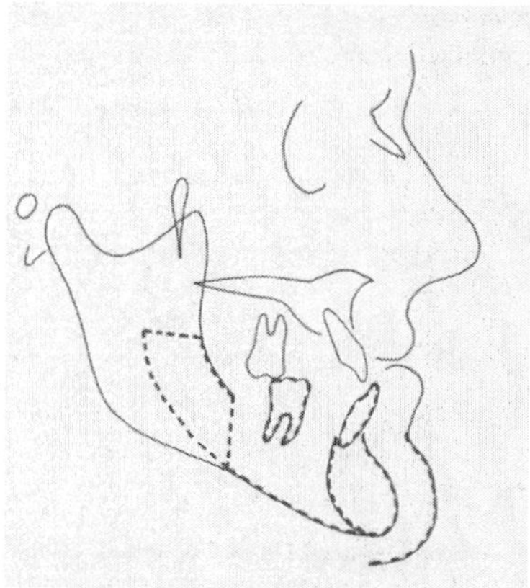

Figure 109. Prediction tracing with overlaid acetate tracing.

The prediction (heavy dashed line) is begun by tracing the distal mandible, the mandibular teeth, and the soft tissue chin on a new piece of tracing acetate overlaid on the tracing. This approximates the actual anatomy (geometry) of the distal mandible, which will be repositioned at surgery. (Figure 109)

The prediction is moved backward on the tracing to achieve the ideal occlusal relations and the stable structures, including the proximal mandible, are traced. The relations of the proximal and distal ramus segments are noted in the body area laterally and in the anterior border area of the ascending ramus (see arrows). After these relationship are noted, accurately determined amounts of bone can be removed in these areas. These relations are important in planning for the surgery to prevent distal rotation of the proximal mandibular segment and the relapse that is related to such rotation. (Figure 110)

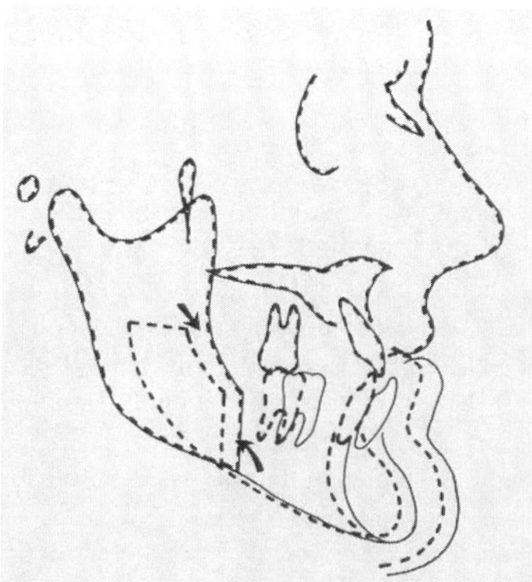

Figure 110. Prediction tracing moved backward.

The need for and details of reduction genioplasty are planned by using both clinical considerations and cephalometric soft tissue relations. Both anteroposterior and vertical relations are considered.

Subnasale perpendicular and the vertical facial soft tissue referent are constructed on the prediction. The soft tissues move approximately 0.8 mm for every 1.0 mm of bony repositioning when a properly done reduction genioplasty is performed. In this instance it is determined that the bony chin is to be repositioned 10 mm superiorly and 7 mm posteriorly to optimize the soft tissue chin position. The desired position of the bony chin is marked on the prediction with crossing vertical and horizontal lines and both the existing bony and soft tissue chins are erased from the prediction. (Figure 111)

The reduction genioplasty is added to the prediction by moving the prediction inferiorly and anteriorly relative to the tracing until the bony chin on the tracing lies in the desired position as indicated by the vertical and horizontal reference lines previously placed. The bony chin is traced in this position on the prediction. (Figure 112)

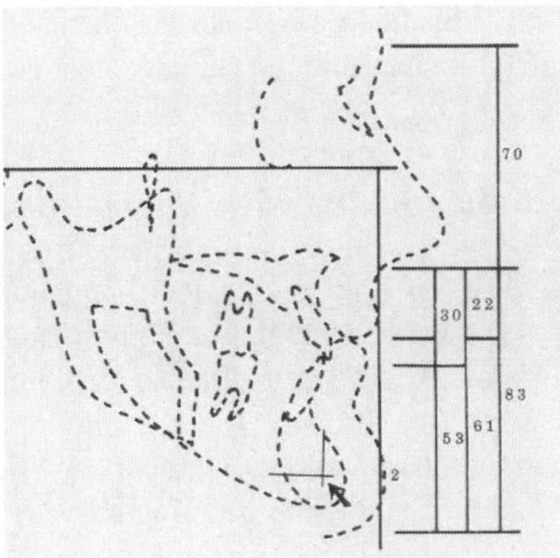

Figure 111. Prediction tracing with planned reduction genioplasty.

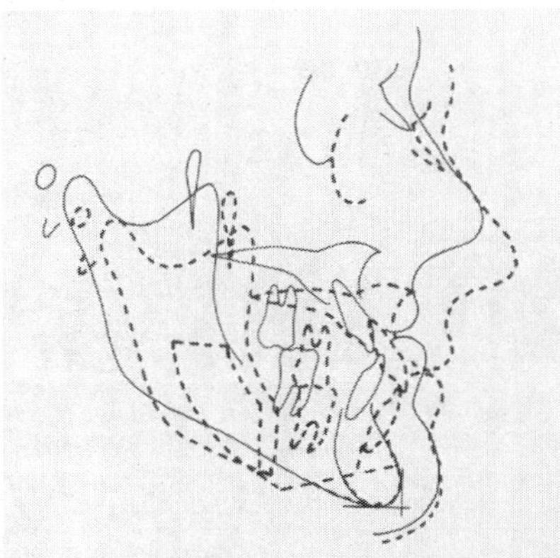

Figure 112. Prediction tracing with positioned bony chin.

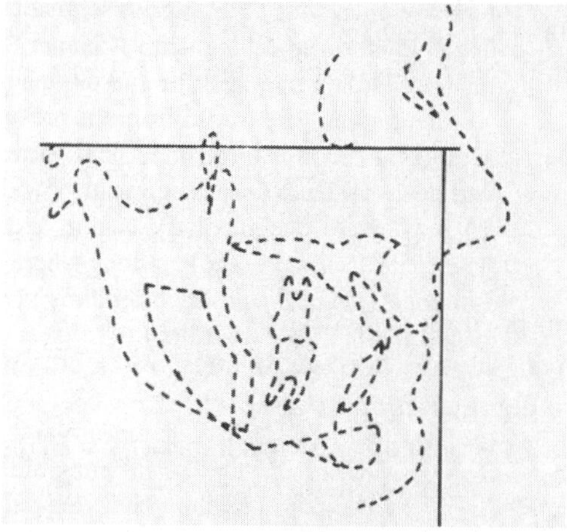

Figure 113. Prediction tracing completed.

The completed prediction is illustrated. The planned changes of the genioplasty must be compatible with both the clinical findings and the patient's desires. (Figure 113)

Superior Repositioning of the Maxilla with Augmentation Genioplasty

All structures are traced from the presurgical cephalometric radiograph. When segmentalization is to be done, it is particularly important to include the anterior and posterior teeth in each segment. Two +'s are made on this tracing 35 mm and 25 above the maxillary canine and first molar respectively (see arrows). These are in the precise locations where the vertical referents are made and the horizontal lateral maxillary osteotomy is done at the time of surgery. This will be called the tracing (solid line). (Figure 114)

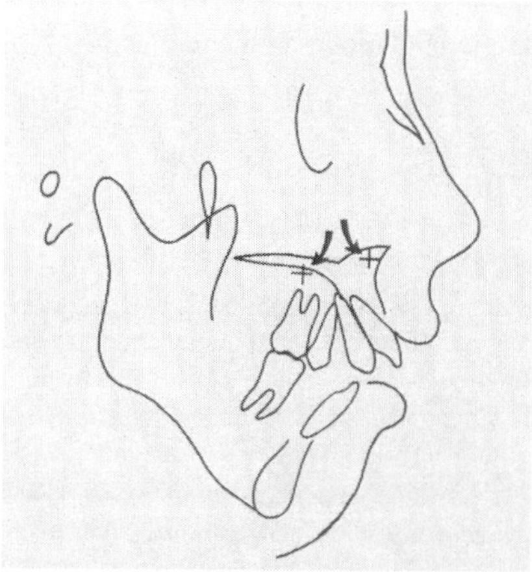

Figure 114. Prediction tracing with vertical referents.

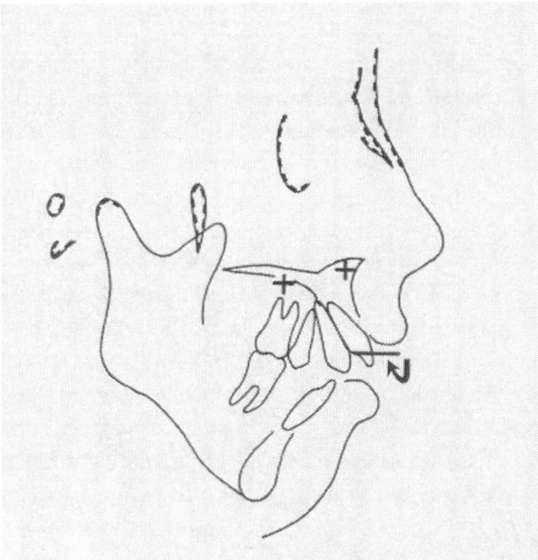

Figure 115. Prediction tracing with prediction arrow and vertical and horizontal skeletal referent.

The prediction (heavy dashed line) is begun by tracing the stable structures that are not to be moved at surgery and the articular surface of the condyle on a new piece of tracing acetate overlaid on the tracing. In addition the two +'s are transferred from the tracing to the prediction to mark the location where the vertical and horizontal skeletal referents will be placed on the maxilla at surgery. The desired vertical location of the upper incisor edge is indicated on the prediction. (see arrow in Figure 115)

The prediction is rotated clockwise about the condyle head, in effect auto-rotating the mandible, until the mandibular incisors are positioned 2 mm superior to the horizontal line previously drawn to indicate the desired vertical position of the maxillary incisors (see arrow). The mandible, mandibular teeth, and soft tissue chin are traced onto the prediction while this superimposition is held. (Figure 116)

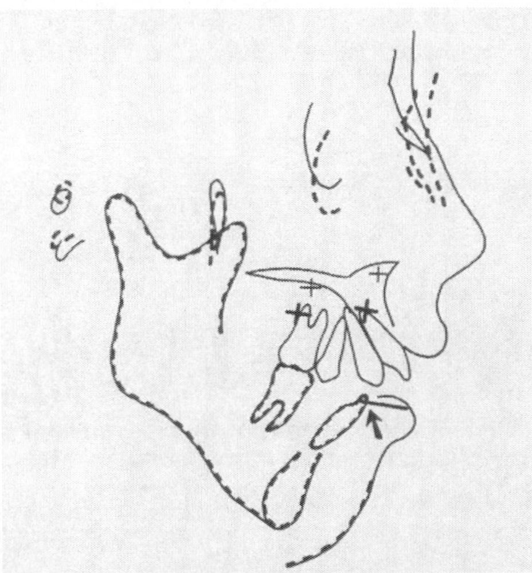

Figure 116. Prediction tracing rotated clockwise about the condyle head.

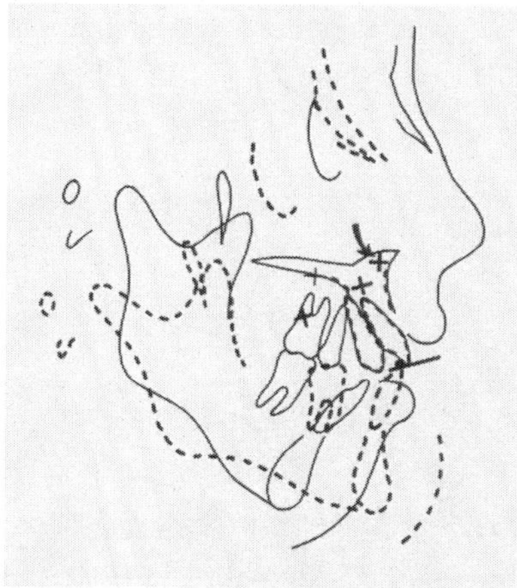

Figure 117. Prediction tracing with ideal maxillary anterior occlusal relationship.

The prediction is repositioned on the tracing such that the maxillary dentition is placed into an ideal occlusal relationship with the mandibular dentition. When segmental procedures are done, this will require two superimpositions—one for the anterior segment and one for the posterior segment. First, the anterior segment, canine through central incisor, is placed. The teeth and anterior maxilla are traced and the referent mark (+) above the canine is transferred to the prediction (see arrow). (Figure 117)

Next the posterior segment, second premolar, and molar are placed into their ideal occlusal relations. The teeth are traced in this position and the referent mark (+) above the first molar is transferred to the prediction (see arrow). When whole arch superior repositioning is done, the step above is eliminated and the new position of the maxillary dentition and the maxilla, including both skeletal referents are traced. The actual changes in the skeletal referents indicate the precise size of the lateral wall ostectomy (horizontal referents) and the required antero-posterior repositioning of the maxilla (vertical referents) that is to be achieved at surgery. In the case of whole-arch maxillary superior repositioning these referents are definitive. (Figure 118)

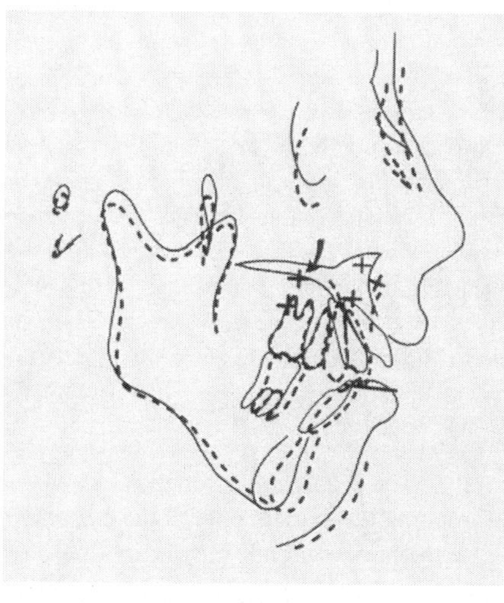

Figure 118. Prediction tracing with ideal maxillary posterior occlusal relationship.

Inferior Repositioning of the Maxilla or Maxillary Advancement

The surgery is to be a whole-arch inferior repositioning of the maxilla. All structures are traced from the presurgical cephalometric radiograph obtained in mandibular rest position. It is essential that the rest position radiograph be used so that accurate determination of the upper tooth-to-lip relation and the true upper lip length can be made and will be reflected in the final result. Two + 's are made on the tracing 35 mm and 25 mm above the canine and the first molar teeth respectively (see arrows). These are indicative of the location of the vertical referents that will be made at surgery and the location of the lateral maxillary wall osteotomy. This will be called the tracing (solid line). (Figure 119)

When a prediction tracing for maxillary advancement is to be done, the usual cephalometric radiograph with the teeth in occlusion is used. All other steps in doing the prediction are the same, in principle, as those illustrated for inferior maxillary repositioning. When the preexisting vertical facial relations are normal and no change is desired in these, no rotation of the mandible and occlusal plane is desired. In this instance that step is omitted. (Figure 120)

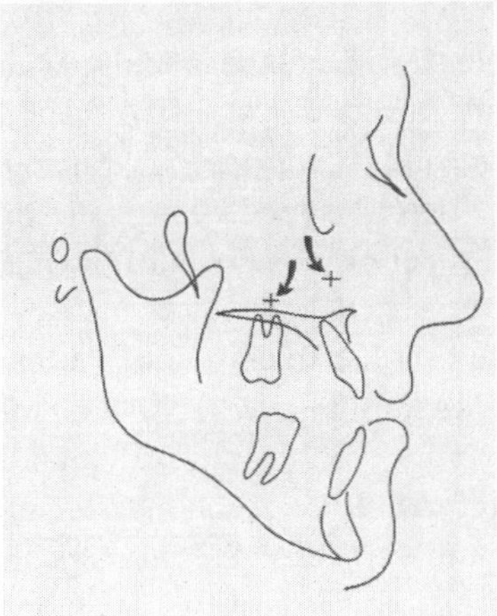

Figure 119. Prediction tracing with vertical referents.

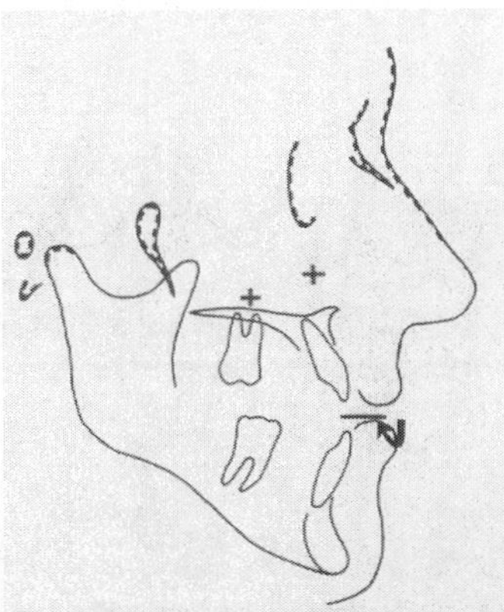

Figure 120. Prediction tracing for maxillary advancement.

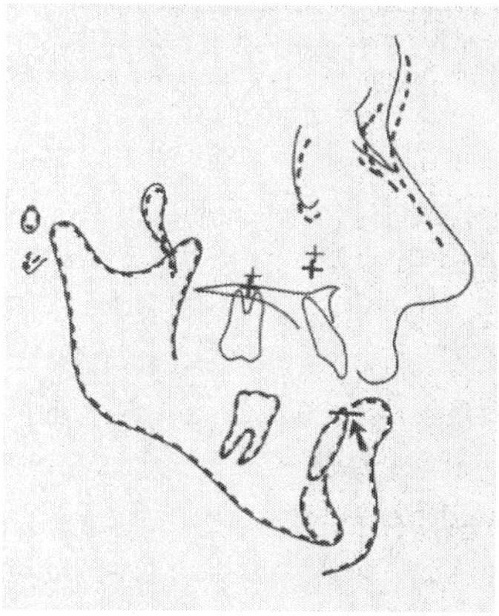

Figure 121. Prediction tracing with horizontal vertical line.

The prediction (heavy dashed line) is begun by tracing the stable structures, including the articular surface of the condyle, on a new piece of acetate overlaid on the tracing. The two +'s placed on the tracing are transferred to the prediction, and a horizontal line is made to indicate the desired vertical position of the upper incisor edge (see arrow). (Figure 121)

The prediction is rotated clockwise on the tracing, with the condyle as the center of rotation, in effect autorotating the mandible, until the mandibular incisors are positioned 2 mm above the horizontal referent line (see arrow). The mandible, mandibular dentition, and associated soft tissues are traced onto the prediction while this superimposition is held. For maxillary advancement when no superior movement of the maxilla is desired, these structures are traced as part of the stable structures. (Figure 122)

The prediction is repositioned on the tracing until the maxillary teeth of the tracing are placed into a Class I occlusion with normal overbite and overjet with the mandibular teeth on the prediction. The maxilla, maxillary teeth, and referent lines (+'s) are traced onto the prediction in this position. The referent lines in the maxilla are used to determine the amount of the maxillary repositioning, both vertically and anteroposteriorly, required to achieve the desired esthetic result. This information is necessary to determine the proper size and shape of the inter-positional bone grafts at surgery. (Figure 123)

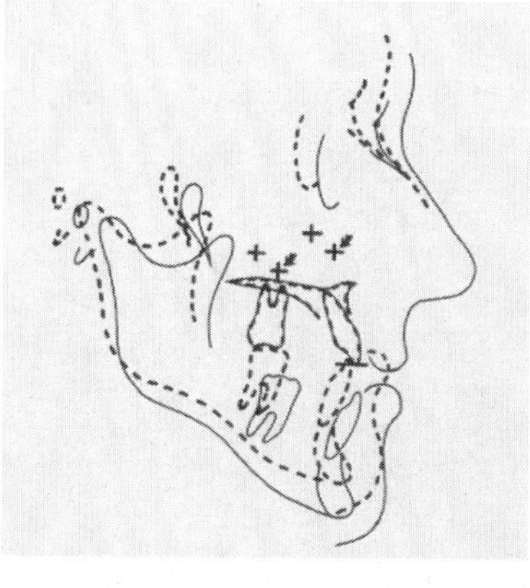

Figure 122. Prediction tracing rotated clockwise.

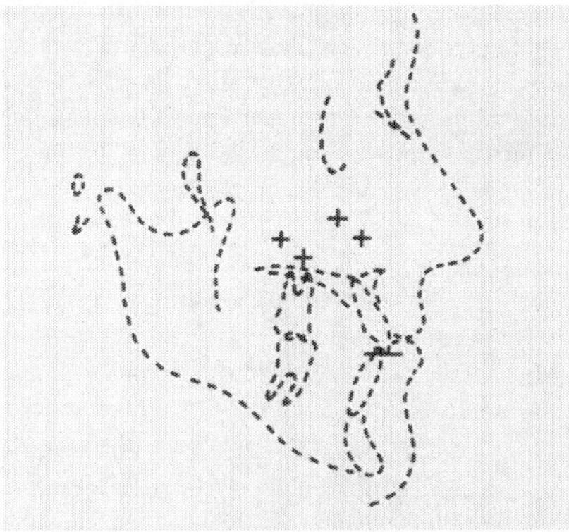

Figure 123. Prediction tracing with ideal Class I occlusal relationship.

Considerations for genioplasty may be necessary, and when this is so, they are essentially the same as described previously. After completing any necessary genioplasty, the soft tissues are added as described. The completed prediction is illustrated.

Simultaneous Two-Jaw Surgery

The most frequently done simultaneous two-jaw procedure is superior repositioning of the maxilla with mandibular advancement. Importantly all simultaneous two-jaw procedures are combinations of the aforementioned procedures. (Figure 124)

All structures are traced from the presurgical cephalometric radiograph. Two +'s are made on this tracing 35 mm and 25 mm above the maxillary canines and first molars respectively (see arrows), and the mandibular functional occlusal plane is traced. This will be called the tracing (solid line). (Figure 125)

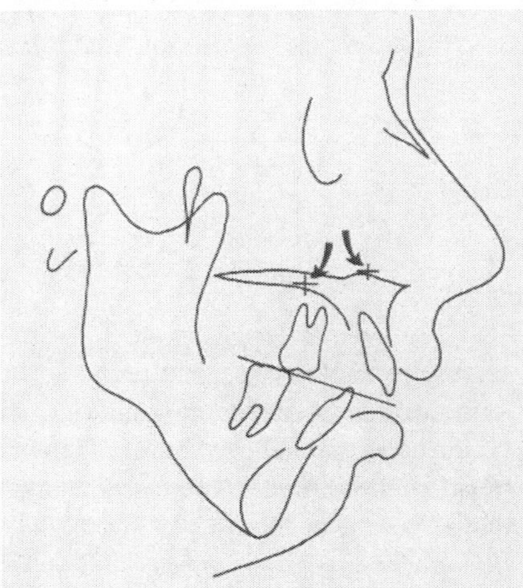

Figure 124. Prediction tracing for two jaw surgery.

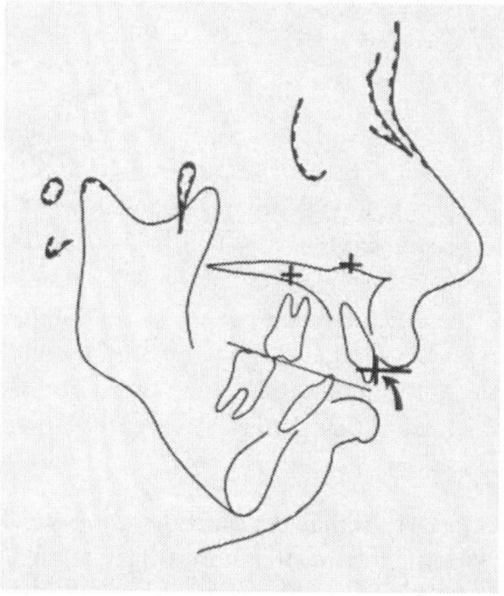

Figure 125. Prediction tracing with mandibular functional occlusal plane.

The prediction (heavy dashed line) is begun by tracing the stable structures that are not to be moved at surgery, including the articular surface of the condyle on a new piece of acetate overlaid on the tracing. The two +'s are transferred from the tracing to the prediction to mark where the referent lines will be placed on the lateral wall of the maxilla at surgery. A horizontal line is made on {he prediction to mark the desired vertical location of the upper incisor edge and crossed by a vertical line on the prediction to reference the present anteroposterior position of the upper incisor to help in judging the amount of advancement of the maxilla (see arrow). (Figure 127)

The prediction is rotated clockwise with the condyle as the center of rotation until the mandibular functional occlusal plane lies one mm above the intersection of the vertical and horizontal upper incisor referents. The proximal portion of the mandible and the mandibular functional occlusal plane are traced onto the prediction while this superimposition is held. The desired vertical position of the dentition has now been established. (Figure 128)

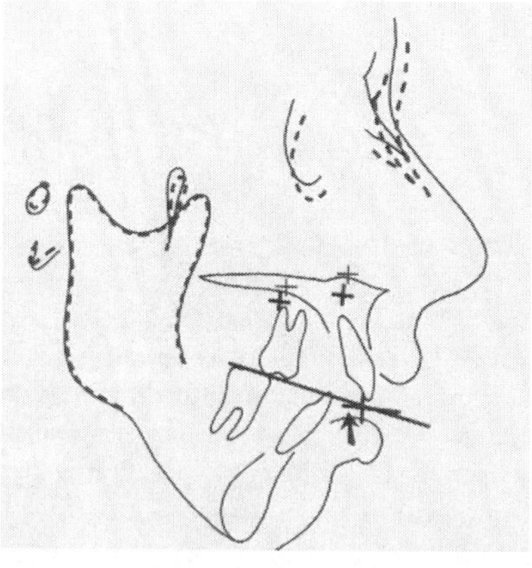

Figure 127. Prediction tracing with horizontal line.

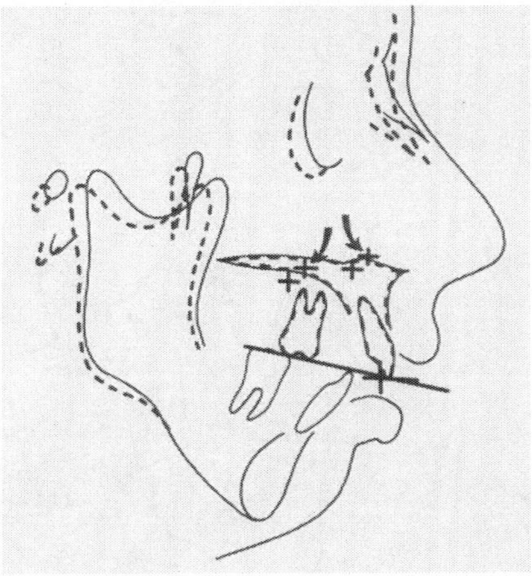

Figure 128. Prediction tracing with anticlockwise rotation.

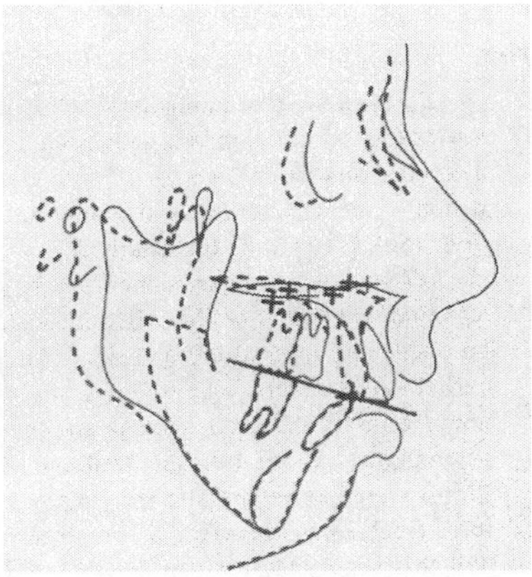

Figure 128. Prediction tracing with maxillary teeth placed according to the occlusal plane of the prediction.

The prediction is repositioned on the tracing until the maxillary teeth of the tracing are placed in the normal relation to the occlusal plane of the prediction. In addition, the anteroposterior location of the repositioned maxilla must be determined. This is predicated primarily on facial esthetics, nasal prominence, para-nasal configuration, alar base anatomy, and upper lip drape (nasolabial angle). The amount of anterior maxillary repositioning is based on the amount of change desired in the aforementioned structures and is determined by observing the anterior movement of both the incisor edge and the superior referent marks. Once the desired vertical and anteroposterior changes are produced by repositioning the prediction, this superimposition is maintained and the maxillary teeth, maxilla, and referent marks are traced onto the prediction. (When the maxillary surgery is to be segmental, the above procedure will require separate repositioning for the anterior and posterior segments as described previously in the section in this chapter on segmental superior repositioning.) The skeletal referent lines (+'s) are essential because they determine the specific size of the lateral maxillary ostectomies (horizontal referents) and the amount of anteroposterior repositioning (vertical referents). (Figure 128)

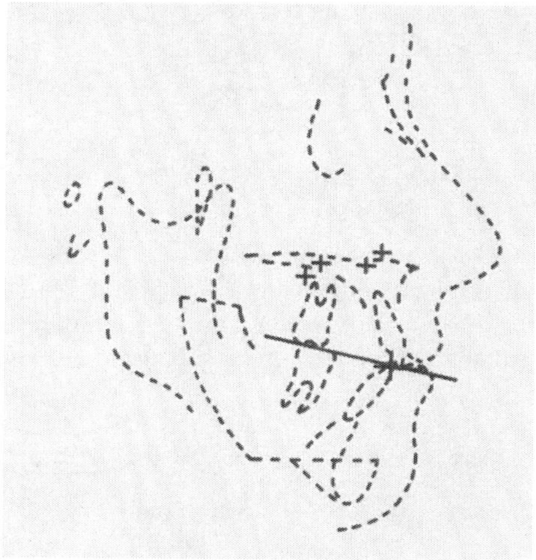

Figure 129. Prediction tracing with advanced distal mandible.

The prediction is now moved backward relative to the tracing along the occlusal plane until the mandibular dentition on the tracing is in the desired occlusal relation with the maxillary dentition on the prediction. This advances the distal mandible; the mandibular teeth and soft tissue chin are traced on the prediction in this position. The tracing of the distal mandible approximates the actual anatomy (geometry) that will be repositioned at surgery. In this way the relations of the proximal and distal ramus segments can be noted so that the proper relations of the intraosseous holes and wires can be achieved at surgery to control the proximal segment and condyle position. (Figure 129)

The soft tissue of the nose and upper lip are traced onto the prediction as described under orthodontic surgical tracing. The soft tissue chin relations are studied, and a determination is made with regard to the need for and, if necessary, the magnitude of an augmentation genioplasty.

This is done as described in the section in this chapter on mandibular advancement. When needed, the genioplasty is added to the prediction. The finished prediction is illustrated.

Definitive Model Surgery and Surgical Occlusal Splint Construction

The definitive model surgery is performed on models obtained shortly before surgery, after it has been determined by feasibility model surgery that the patient is ready for surgery, and is done on either a Class II, type 1 articulator (arbitrary hinge type) or a Class II, type III articulator (anatomic, adjustable type), depending on the specific type of surgery that is to be performed [24].

The definitive model surgery is done for various purposes depending on the specific type of orthognathic surgical procedure that is to be done. The reasons for performing definitive model surgery include (1) to determine the magnitude and direction of skeletal movements, (2) to determine the size and shape of the osteotomies, especially interdental, (3) to provide a vehicle for surgical splint construction, and (4) to provide a comparative referent to the occlusal result actually achieved as noted on release of intermaxillary fixation. It is ideal if the definitive model surgery is maintained as part of the patient's records or photographed. When complications occur, these records are useful and can be compared with the occlusion that existed on release of intermaxillary fixation or exists during any phase of postsurgical orthodontics.

Mandibular Advancement

Any type of articulator is satisfactory for performing the definitive model surgery for mandibular advancement. The details of skeletal movement and intraosseous wire placement are best determined from the surgical cephalometric prediction tracing. The primary purpose of the definitive model surgery is to hold the models in the desired relation (that is, the relationship that is to be obtained at surgery) during the construction of the surgical occlusal splint. On these models it is important to establish a satisfactory Class I occlusion, overbite, overjet, and transverse relation that will permit uncomplicated postsurgical orthodontic finishing of the occlusion. (Figure 130, 131)

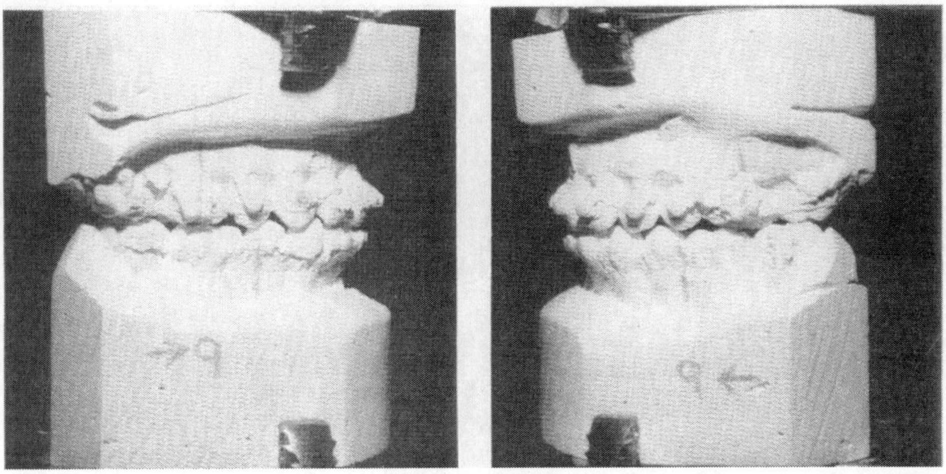

Figure 130. Articulator with mounted models.

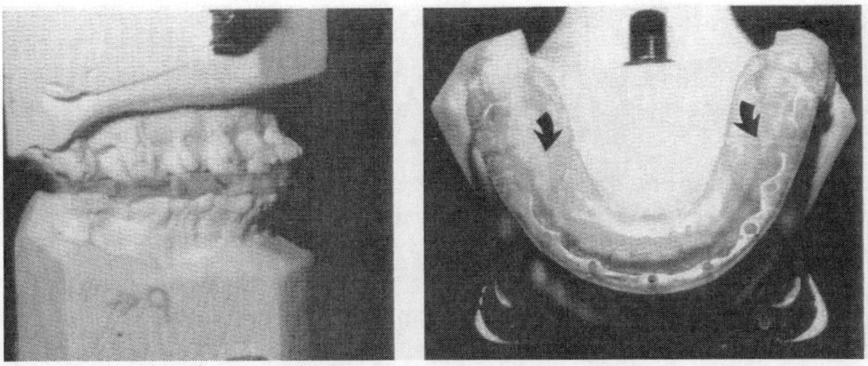

Figure 131. Models with occlusal splint.

It the occlusion is such that as a result of the presurgical orthodontics the models can unequivocally be positioned into an optimal occlusion, an occlusal splint need not be used. This is often not the case, and an occlusal splint is used. There is no overcorrection either anteroposteriorly or vertically. Since the surgical occlusal splint is to be secured to the mandibular dentition by circummandibular wires at the time of surgery, grooves are made in the splint between the premolars and molars (arrows) so that the circummandibular wires are located between the maxillary teeth. This eliminates occlusal interferences, since these wires pass over the occlusal aspect of the splint. The splint is not extended distally beyond the terminal molars; doing so reduces the space available for the patient to drink the blended diet during intermaxillary fixation. Moreover, this extension will generally result in occlusal interferences after the release of intermaxillary fixation, when the splint is left wired to the mandible, during the period of jaw physiotherapy. Likewise the maxillary occlusal interdigitations are definite, but shallow, to preclude occlusal interferences when the intermaxillary fixation is released and the patient begins to initiate jaw function (physiotherapy) with the splint left secured to the mandible.

Mandibular Setback

The definitive model surgery and surgical occlusal splint construction are identical to that described for mandibular advancement, except that the buccal and lingual notches in the splint are located between the canines are premolars. When skeletal intermaxiallary fixation is employed, the circummandibular wires are placed more anteriorly with setback of the mandible.

Segmental Superior Repositioning of the Maxilla

With superior repositioning of the maxilla without segmentalization, a carefully done surgical cephalometric prediction tracing provides accurate and essential information for surgery. When segmental superior repositioning of the maxilla is to be done, as for the Class II deformity with open bite, the definitive model surgery is performed on an anatomic articulator (type II, Class III). The models are made from impressions taken shortly before surgery, are trimmed to simulate the actual skeletal anatomy of the maxilla, and are mounted on the articulator by a face-bow transfer. (Figure 132)

The mounted models are marked as follows:

1. The tooth roots adjacent to all interdental osteotomies or ostectomies are drawn on the models in their existing locations as determined from the radiographs.
2. Vertical referent lines (perpendicular to Frankfort horizontal plane) are drawn from the mounting ring of the maxillary model to the first molar and canine teeth bilaterally, and the skeletal midline is similarly referenced. These lines extend onto the mandibular dentition.
3. Parallel vertical referent lines are drawn on both sides of the proposed interdental osteotomies.

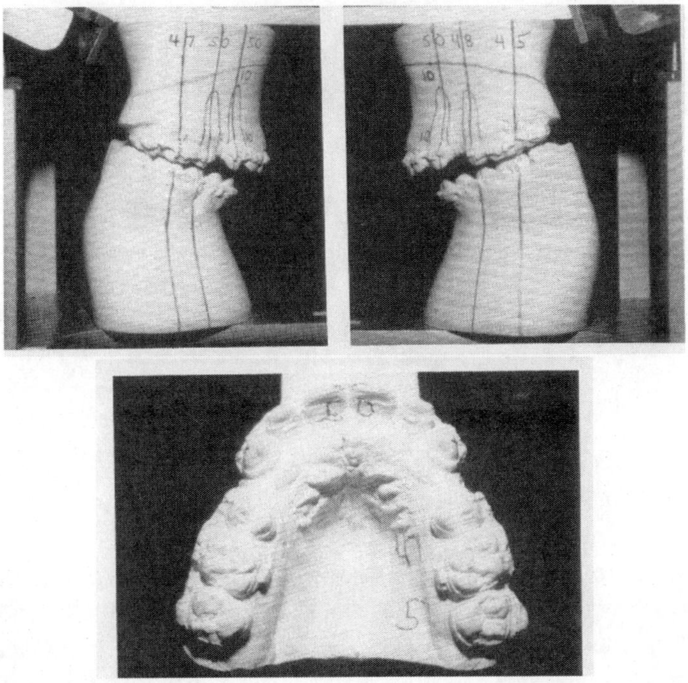

Figure 132. Models for superior repositioning of maxilla.

A horizontal line is drawn on the models approximately 35 mm above the maxillary canine cusp tips and 25 mm above the maxillary first molar cusp tips. This will closely simulate the inferior location of the lateral maxillary wall osteotomy to be made at surgery. (Figure 132)

The following measurements are made and recorded on the models:

1. The distance between the two parallel vertical referent lines adjacent to any proposed interdental ostectomy
2. The distance from maxillary mounting ring to the first molar and canine-cusp tips bilaterally and to the incisal edge of the central incisors
3. The intercanine, interpremolar, and intermolar distances

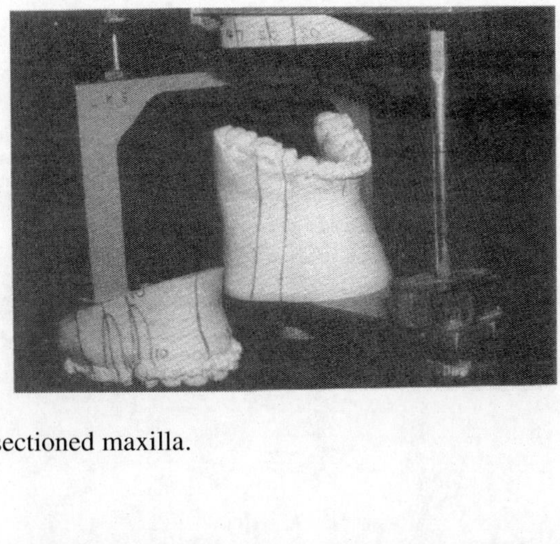

Figure 133. Models with sectioned maxilla.

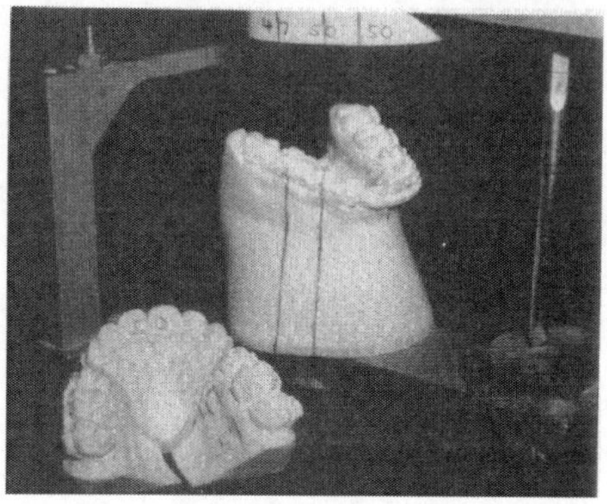

Figure 134. Maxillary model with interdental osteotomy cuts.

The maxilla is sectioned from its base along the line drawn on the maxillary model that indicates the location of the inferior osteotomy to be performed at surgery. Next, plaster is removed from the superior aspect of the maxillary base in excess of the amount that the maxillary segments are to be superiorly repositioned so that a layer of soft wax can be applied to this base for the subsequent temporary placement of the maxillary segments. (Figure 133)

The indicated interdental osteotomies or ostectomies are done on the maxillary model to separate it into the indicated three or four segments. Care is taken in performing these to avoid cutting through or into the tooth roots. Doing so will ultimately result in either an inability to achieve the indicated segmental movements or actual injury to the tooth roots adjacent to the interdental osteotomy or ostectomy sites at surgery. (Figure 134)

The anterior maxillary segment is placed into its optimal occlusal relation with the mandibular teeth and lightly sticky waxed to the lower teeth in this position. The articulator is closed, and the change in the anterior vertical relation (distance from central incisor edge to mounting ring) is measured to obtain the predetermined amount of superior repositioning (decrease in distance from central incisor edge to mounting ring) of the anterior maxillary teeth. The specific amount of vertical movement has been previously determined, on an esthetic basis, to normalize upper tooth-to-lip relations and achieve optimal upper tooth-to-lip esthetics. Once the articulator has been closed the appropriate amount, the incisal guide pin is locked in this position and the anterior segment is rejoined to the base with soft wax. (Figure 135)

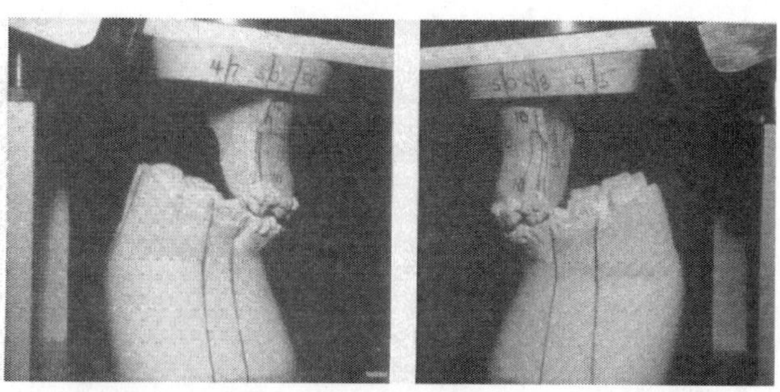

Figure 135: Anterior maxillary segment placed in optimal occlusion with mandibular teeth.

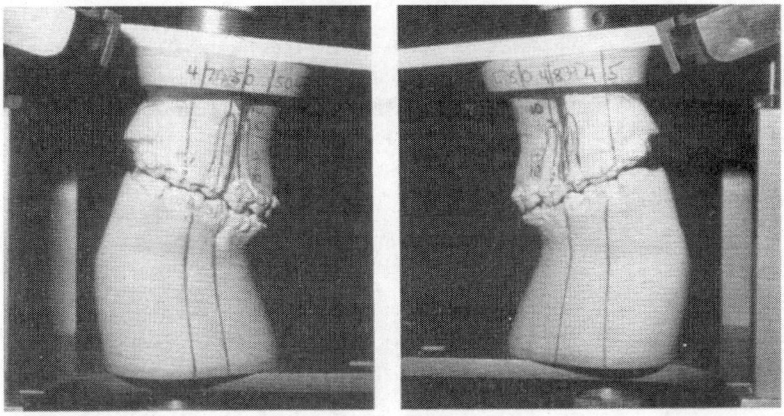

Figure 136. Properly positioned anterior and posterior segments.

The posterior maxillary segments are positioned to achieve the best possible occlusion and rejoined to the base with soft wax. This may require some additional removal of interdental plaster but must be done without cutting into the tooth roots. Once the maxillary segments are all properly positioned to achieve both the best possible occlusion and the indicated amount of superior repositioning, they are secured rigidly to one another and to the superior base with a heavy application of sticky wax.(Figure 136)

The actual magnitude of the anterior or posterior movements of the segments are noted from the changes in the vertical referent lines. The precise magnitude of the lateral maxillary wall ostectomies are measured in the molar and canine areas and recorded on the models. This is done by remeasuring the vertical distances from canine and molar cusps to the maxillary mounting ring and subtracting these values from those made and recorded before doing the surgery on the models. Importantly, the magnitude of superior repositioning in the incisor area, canine and first molar areas are variable and are best determined by carefully done model surgery. (Figure 137)

The magnitude of the intermolar, interpremolar, and intercanine change is measured and recorded, since the magnitude of change (palatal expansion or constriction) will determine the need for either midpalatal ostectomy or palatal soft tissue relaxing incisions.

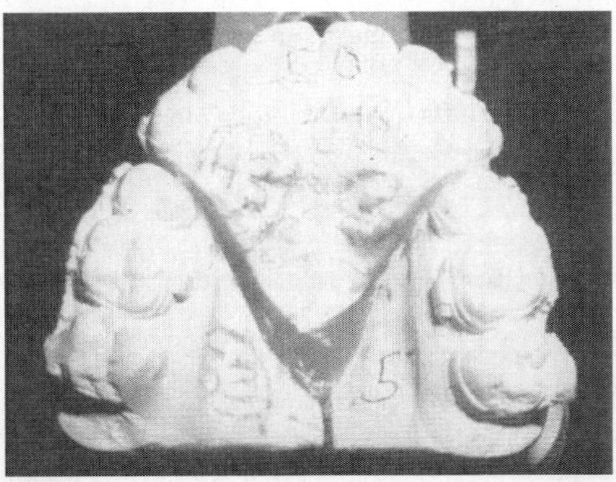

Figure 137. Recording of the magnitude of osteotomy cuts on the models.

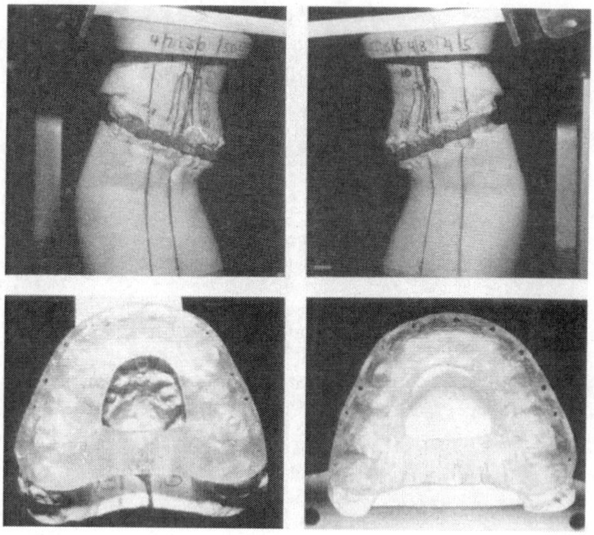

Figure 138. Models with acrylic occlusal splint.

The acrylic surgical occlusal splint is now constructed on the models. The maxillary dentition is maximally interdigitated into the splint to permit optimal positioning of the maxillary segments at the time of surgery. When these inter-digitations are not discrete, there is a tendency for the segments to be arbitrarily tipped either buccally or palatally at the actual time of surgery. (Figure 138)

The splint does not extend past the terminal molars. The mandibular occlusal interdigitations are definite, but shallow, to preclude occlusal interferences when the intermaxillary fixation is released and the patient begins to initiate jaw function (physiotherapy) with the splint left secured to the maxilla. Importantly, this is nor to be a functional splint from the standpoint that the patient can masticate with it in place. Rather, it is to permit hinge-axis closure of the mandible so that the patient's occlusion can be checked periodically after release of intermaxillary fixation to make certain the surgical result is stable.

A heavy transpalatal acrylic bar is used to afford transverse stabilization. This is relieved 2 to 3 mm so that it does not encroach upon the palatal mucosa, since this will result in compromise of the essential palatal vascular pedicle and probable avascular necrosis of the segments. This relief must be 2 to 3 mm more than the size of the lateral maxillary wall ostectomies in the molar area when the maxillary total subapical procedure, which leaves the palate at the presurgical level, is to be done.

Inferior Repositioning of the Maxilla or Maxillary Advancement

When whole-arch (one piece) inferior repositioning or advancement of the maxilla is to be done, the surgical cephalometric prediction tracing done as described earlier, will provide the essential information regarding the details of surgical repositioning, and definitive model surgery need not be performed on an anatomic articulator. Thus in these instances the model surgery and splint construction may be performed on any type of articulator. (Figure 139)

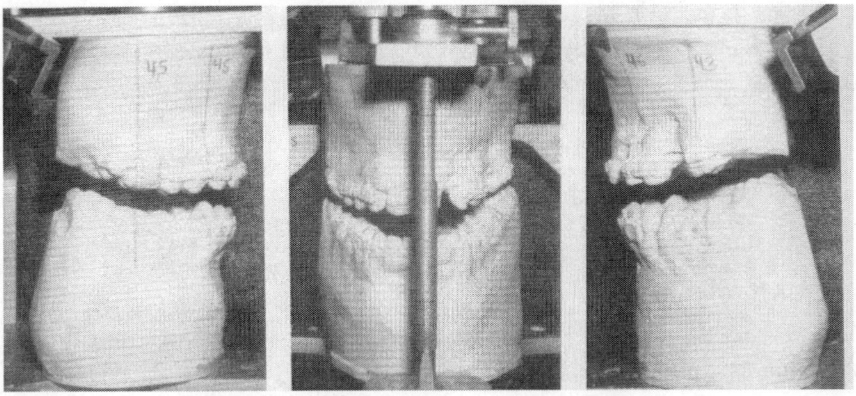

Figure 139. Anatomic articulator with mounted models.

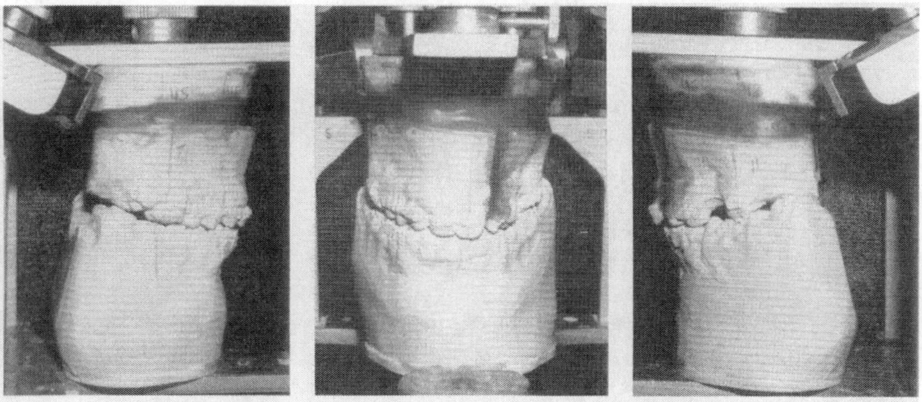

Figure 140. Anatomic articulator with mounted models having markings.

When segmentalization of the maxilla is to be done with inferior repositioning or advancement of the maxilla with variable amounts of repositioning of the segments, definitive model surgery is best done on an anatomic articulator. This allows optimal precision in planning the details of skeletal surgical movement and bone grafting.

The models are trimmed to simulate the actual anatomy and mounted on the articulator by a face-bow transfer. A bite registration is made such that its thickness anteriorly is equal to the distance that the anterior maxillary teeth are planned, on an esthetic basis, to be inferiorly repositioned (illustrated), while a normal occlusal registration is used for maxillary advancement. The models are marked, and measurements are made and recorded on the models as previously described for superior repositioning of the maxilla. (Figure 140)

The maxillary model is sectioned from its base at the level that the actual lateral wall osteotomies will be made at surgery. The maxilla is segmentalized as indicated, placed into the best possible occlusal relation with the mandibular dentition, and either lightly sticky waxed together at this time or stabilized with soft wax to the superior base.

After the optimal occlusion is achieved, the maxillary segments are secured to the base and to one another with a heavy application of sticky wax. The precise magnitude of vertical change in the piriform and molar areas is then measured bilaterally. These are duplicated at surgery via bone grafting. Note that the left and right sides may require bone grafts that are highly variable in size. The antero-posterior and transverse relations are also noted. The occlusal splint is constructed with a heavy transpalatal bar as described earlier for superior repositioning of the maxilla.

Simultaneous Two-Jaw Surgery

With simultaneous repositioning of the maxilla and advancement of the mandible as single units (that is, no segmentalization) any articulator is adequate to perform the model surgery and construct the surgical occlusal splint, providing a detailed surgical cephalometric prediction tracing is done to determine the details of the surgery so that the planned or indicated movements at surgery can be properly determined to produce the desired esthetic and occlusal results. (Figure 141)

When segmentalization of the maxilla is to be done in concert with either mandibular advancement or setback, as is commonly performed in the Class II or III deformity with open bite, an anatomic articulator is preferable. The identical sequence of model mounting and marking, as described for superior repositioning of the maxilla, is done. In addition, the approximate location of the inferior border of the mandible is indicated on the mandibular model base from measurements made on the cephalometric radiograph. A vertical referent is made in the mid-symphysis area.

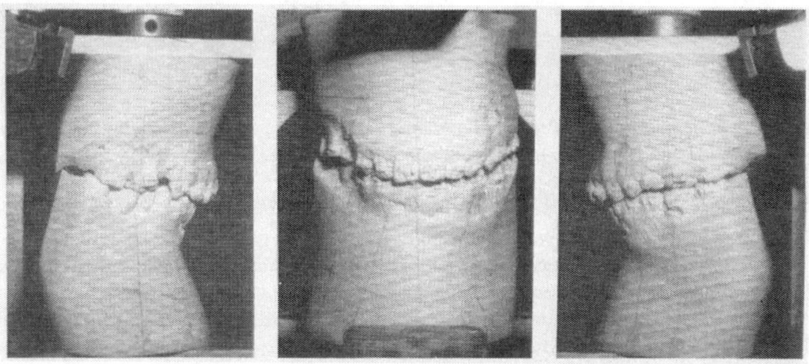

Figure 141. Anatomic articulator with mounted models.

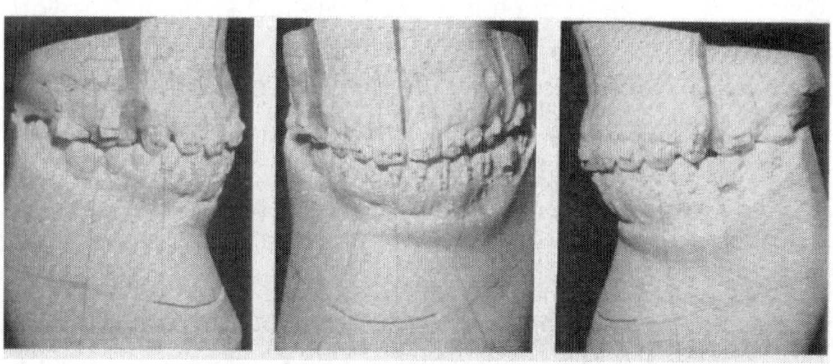

Figure 142. Anatomic articulator with mounted models with superior segmental maxillary repositioning.

The maxilla is removed along a line approximating the level of the inferior aspect of the osteotomy at surgery. The maxilla is segmentalized as previously described in this chapter for superior segmental repositioning of the maxilla. (Figure 142)

The maxillary segments are placed into the best possible occlusion with the mandibular teeth and are stabilized with soft wax or a light application of sticky wax between the maxillary and mandibular teeth. Once their optimal occlusion is achieved with the mandible, they are consolidated into a single unit with a heavy application of sticky wax. Once the pieces of the maxilla have been thus rejoined, this "single piece" maxilla is now removed from the mandibular base and repositioned. (Figure 143)

Predicted on the desired anteroposterior relation, vertical maxillary incisor relation, and desired occlusal plane orientation, the maxillary segment is repositioned as a unit, stabilized with soft wax to the maxillary base, and studied. Great care is taken not to cause any asymmetric repositioning and to maintain or correct the midline.

If an intermediate splint is to be used, it is constructed between the repositioned maxillary segments and the mandibular component that has not been sectioned free from the articulator. While this intermediate splint does provide both a transverse and an anteroposterior referent and may be helpful in allowing the surgeon to eliminate any interferences to the desired superior repositioning, this splint does not provide any essential information regarding the proper or desired vertical (superior) positioning of the maxilla at surgery. This is because the mobilized maxilla can be placed into the splint, and there is no index, except for the actual model surgery lateral wall referent marks, as to how little or much to autorotate the maxillary-mandibular complex. Thus this splint is not a substitute for the definitive cephalometric prediction tracing and model surgery. (Figure 144)

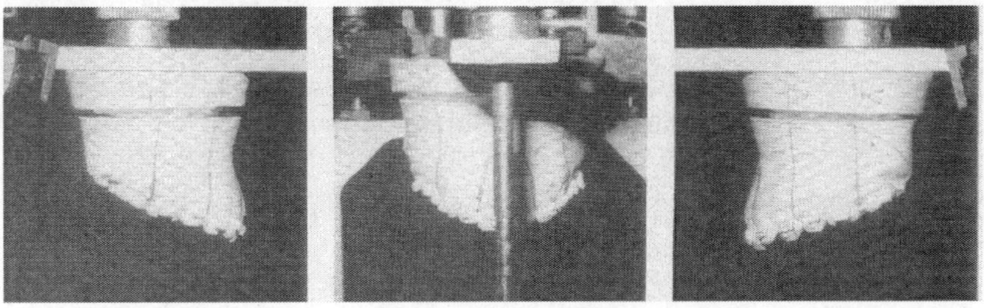

Figure 143. Anatomic articulator with repositioned "single piece" maxilla.

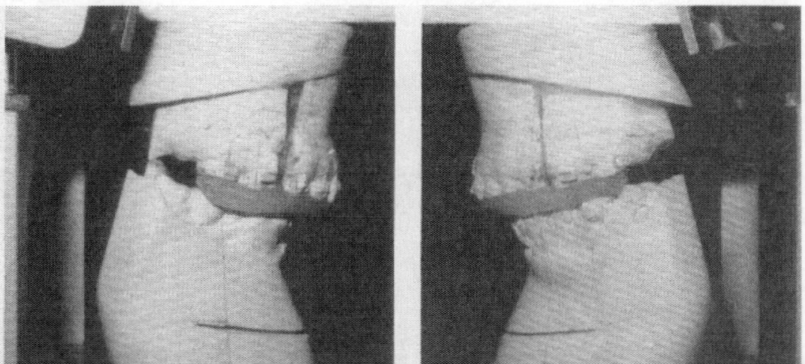

Figure 144. Anatomic articulator with intermediate splint.

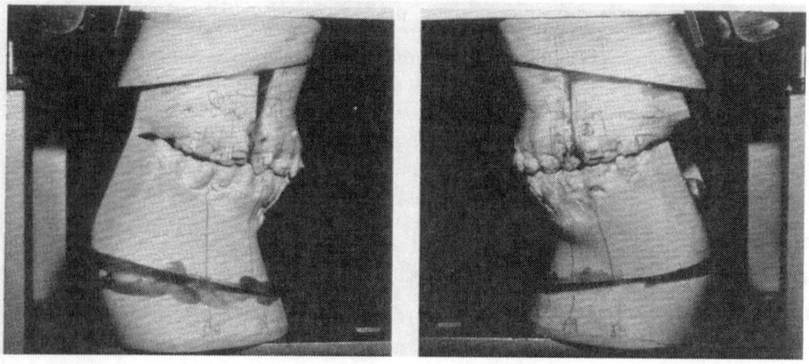

Figure 145. Anatomic articulator with maxillary and mandibular segments attached with sticky wax with their respective bases.

The mandibular component is now removed and repositioned into its ideal occlusal relation with the maxilla. Once it has been manipulated and the final occlusal relations are established, the maxillary and mandibular segments are securely attached to their respective bases with a heavy application of sticky wax. A surgical occlusal splint is constructed as described previously [24]. (Figure 145)

Immediate Presurgical Orthodontic Planning

It is essential that the orthodontist have placed his surgical arch wires at least 4 to 6 weeks prior to the taking of presurgical records. This time span is necessary to ensure that any dental changes caused by insertion of the arch wires are fully manifested and that there is no change between the time of presurgical records and the actual surgical procedure.

Heavy rectangular arch wires, filling as much of the slot as possible, with full engagement are most often used in the maxilla, either as a continuous arch or in segments where this is indicated. In the mandible a similar wire is used where anterior face height is to be decreased (open bites or open-bite tendencies) so as to provide maximum stability since little postoperative mechanotherapy should be required. When the mandibular occlusal plane is to be leveled after surgery (short face height, deep bites), lighter, more resilient wires are advisable. Elastics from the heavy rectangular maxillary arch wire to the lighter mandibular arch wire will rapidly effect postsurgical leveling of the lower arch [51].

Some type of aid to facilitate fixation should be placed on the surgical arch wires prior to surgery. The soldering of numerous small hooks onto the arch wires is a tedious, time-consuming operation, and there is considerable danger of annealing the arch wire. The presence of numerous sharp projections can be very irritating to the lips and cheeks, as well as producing increased oral hygiene problems. The use of attachments, such as sliding surgical ball hooks or Guerin locks, provides sufficient fixation points, considerably reduces the time needed to prepare the arch wires, removes the danger of annealing the arch wires, and allows the same wires to be used postsurgically subsequent to the use of light wires to correct any vertical discrepancies.

Chapter 10

POST-SURGICAL ORTHODONTICS AND RETENTION

***Postsurgical Orthodontic objectives*:** they are generally similar to those considered in finishing a conventional orthodontic case.

1. Attaining final tooth alignment, maximum interdigitation, finalizing torque, and artistic positioning of teeth
2. Attaining ideal overjet/overbite relationship compatible with a mutually protected occlusion where CO equals CR.
3. Establishment of correct root parallelism is important, particularly in segmental cases where the roots of the teeth adjacent to the osteotomy sites [51].

Post surgical orthodontics can begin when the surgeon thinks the healing has reached the point of satisfactory clinical stability. With wire osteosynthesis and maxillomandibular fixation, clinical healing to this level usually requires 6-8 weeks. The first step in postsurgical orthodontics is to remove the splint and stabilizing archwires. These should be removed at the same time by the orthodontist who can immediately make any necessary repairs to the orthodontic appliance. At this time he should superimpose the cephalometric head films taken before surgery, immediately after surgery, and at the release of fixation. Analysis of the changes seen will enable the clinician to identify precisely what surgical change occurred and also the nature and extent of relapse during fixation. This knowledge is vital in planning the postsurgical phase of treatment [2].

During the immediate post fixation period attention should be directed toward rehabilitation procedures. Patients should be instructed to exercise the jaw-opening muscles within painless limits so that they can ultimately return to maximal opening. These exercises should be carried out with the elastics removed if maxillary surgery has been performed. Lateral and protrusive movements should also be practiced as the patient progresses through what is normally a 2- to 3-week exercise period.

Once the splint and stabilizing arch wires have been removed, the orthodontist needs to place working archwires and begin the process of settling the teeth into full occlusion. Typical working wires are 0.016 steel, which are flexible enough to produce the necessary elongation of some teeth. When torque control of maxillary anterior teeth is particularly needed, it may be better to use a flexible rectangular arch wire. If movement of teeth in only lower arch is required then stabilizing arch wires can be retained in upper and a flexible arch wire placed in lower arch. The final step at the first postsurgical appointment is placing the patient on light vertical elastics, to the posterior segments and also to the anterior segment if there is any open bite tendency, in triangular or box formation with only a slight, if any, Class II or Class III vector. The use of these "short" elastics will minimize the tendency to cause molar extrusion and hence open the bite or cause a CO-to-CR discrepancy, while effecting maximum occlusal interdigitation [51] (Figure 146, 147).

The elastics serve two purposes. First they help bring the teeth into a solid occlusion. Equally important, they override the patient's proprioceptive drive toward positioning the mandible in maximum intercuspation so there will not be a tendency to shift into a relationship that is different from the centric relation [2].

By the second appointment, considerable settling typically occurs and it is no longer necessary to wear the box elastics as consistently. They can be omitted while eating and if occlusion has settled properly, can be worn only at night. At this point, small vertical step bends in the working arch wires may be needed to come into occlusion. An important point to be considered during finishing stages is the management of patients who have had transverse expansion of the maxilla at surgery. This expansion is unstable for approximately 6 months. Transverse control can be maintained by using a heavy labial auxiliary wire (36 mil), which is placed in the headgear tubes on molar bands. It should be maintained until arch wire is stiff enough to maintain control of arch form.

Positioners can be used as a final finishing step in postsurgical orthodontics. Compared to routine patients, postsurgical patients may have increased difficulty adapting to these because of two reasons:

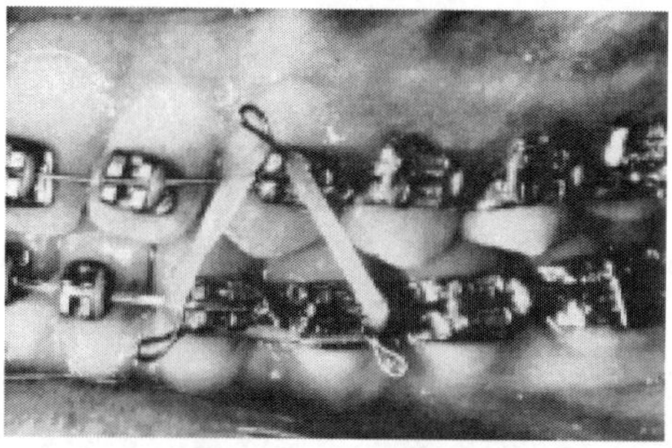

Figure 146. Triangular vertical elastics.

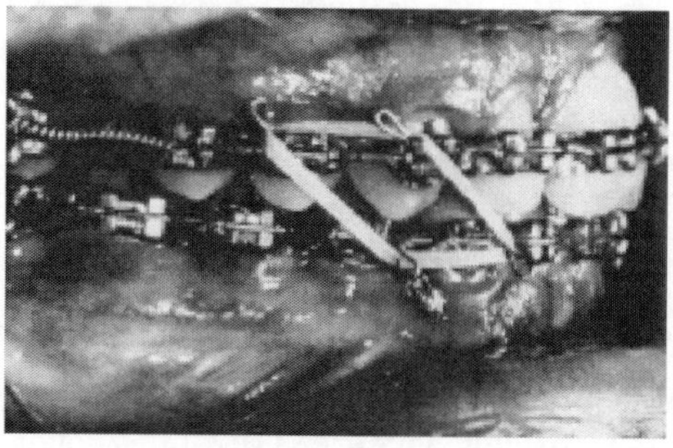

Figure 147. Box elastics with a Class III vector.

1. Some areas of parasthesia may be still be present in the gingiva and/or lips a few months postsurgically
2. Biting force is variably affected by surgery. If bite force decreases the positioner would be less effective.

As a general rule using elastics for final settling of occlusion and then going directly to a retainer is better for surgical patients.

Duration of Postsurgical Orthodontics

The postsurgical treatment time needed to reach such objectives varies according to the type of patient. Those cases in which anterior face height has been decreased (open bites or open-bite tendency) should have been treated virtually to completion prior to surgery. Therefore, a minimum (often no more than 3 to 4 months) of postsurgical treatment should be required. Lengthy postsurgical orthodontic treatment in these cases can lead to compromises in stability and function if the surgical results are disrupted.

In cases that involve increasing lower anterior face height (deep bites), most of the orthodontic tooth movement should be accomplished postsurgically. This may take several months, and there need be little concern about untoward orthodontic effects causing relapse or a compromise of the surgical correction [51].

Retention

It is vital to customize the patient's retention plan according to the characteristics of the original malocclusion and the features of any relapse patterns seen after surgery [51]. The use of a positioner, preferably employing a hinge-axis face-bow recording, has been found to be effective in obtaining close occlusal interdigitation and is thus ideal in cases in which originally there was an open bite. For long-term retention in these cases, removable retainers of the Hawley type can be used in the maxilla.

Care must be taken not to allow retainer wires to pass across the occlusion or through extraction or osteotomy sites. In order to avoid potential occlusal interferences, circumferential ("wrap-around") retainers with additional soldered "C clasps" are advocated. In cases in which relapse may be expected or has already occurred, attachments may be placed on the retainers to counteract these detrimental factors. Small cleats can be welded to the buccal surfaces of the bands of a mandibular canine-to-canine retainer, enabling the patient to wear Class III elastics to small hooks soldered to the buccal wire of a removable maxillary retainer. Similar procedures can involve the use of box elastics for open-bite cases and Class II elastics to a removable lower retainer for a relapsing mandibular advancement.

Deep bite cases should be retained by means of a removable maxillary retainer with a small anterior bite plane if some relapse is expected. A fixed mandibular canine-to-canine retainer provides adequate support to prevent retroclination of the lower incisors.

REFERENCES

[1] Fonseca, R. J. (2000). *Oral and Maxillofacial Surgery*. Vol 2. Philadelphia, W.B. Saunders Company.

[2] Proffit, W. & White, R. (1991). *Surgical Orthodontic Treatment.* St Louis, Mosby - Year Book.

[3] Ackerman, J. L. & Proffit, W. R. (1995). "Communication in orthodontic treatment planning: Bioethical and informed consent issues." *Angle Orthod*, 65, 253.

[4] Graber, T. M. & Swain, B. F. (1985). *Current Orthodontic Concept and Techniques.* St. Louis, Mosby.

[5] Proffit, W. R. & Fields, H. W. (2000). *Contemporary Orthodontics*. St. Louis, Mosby.

[6] Proffit, W, R., Phillips, C., Tulloch, J. F. C. & Medland, P. H. (1992). "Surgical versus orthodontic correction of skeletal Class II malocclusion in adolescents: Effects and Indications." *Int J Adult Orthod Orthognath Surg*, 7, 209 – 220.

[7] Bertolini, F. & Russo, V. (2000). "Pre and postsurgical psychoemotional aspects of the orthognathic surgery patient." *Int J Adult Orthod Orthognath Surg*, 15, 16-23.

[8] Macgregor, F. C. (1970). "Social and psychological implications of dentofacial disfigurement." *Angle Orthod*, 40, 231-233.

[9] Helm, S., Kreiborg, S. & Solow, B. (1985). "Psychosocial implications of malocclusion: a 15 year follow up study in 30 year old Danes." *Am J Orthod*, 87, 110-118.

[10] Shaw, W. C. (1981). "The influence of children's dentofacial appearance on their social attractiveness as judged by peers and lay adults." *Am J Orthod*, 79, 399-415.

[11] Auerbach, S. M., Meredith, J. & Alexander, J. M. (1984). "Psychological factors in adjustment to orthognathic surgery." *J Oral Maxillofac Surg*, 42, 435-440.

[12] Finlay, P. M. & Atkinson, J. M. (1995). "Orthognathic surgery: Patients' expectations, psychological profile and satisfaction with outcome." *Br J Oral Maxillofac Surg*, 33, 9-14.

[13] Kiyak, H. A., West, R. A. & Hohl, T. (1982). "The psychological impact of othognathic surgery: a 9 month follow up." *Am J Orthod*, 81, 404-412.

[14] Flanary, C. M., Barnwell, G. M. & Alexander, J. M. (1985). "Patient perceptions of orthognathic surgery." *Am J Orthod*, 88, 137-145.

[15] Jacobson, A. (1981). "The influence of children's dentofacial appearance on their social attractiveness as judged by peers and lay adults." *Am J Orthod*, 79, 399-415.

[16] Heldt, L. (1982). "Psychological and social aspects of orthognathic treatment." *Am J Orthod*, 82, 318-324.
[17] Kiyak, H. A., Hohl, T. & West, R. A. (1984). "Psychologic changes in orthognathic surgery patients: a 24 month follow up." *J Oral Maxillofac Surg*, 42, 506-512.
[18] Olson, R. E. & Laskin, D. M. (1980). "Expectations of patients from orthognathic surgery." *J Oral Surg*, 38, 283.
[19] Bell, W. H., Proffit, W. R. & White, R. P. (1985). *Surgical Correction of Dentofacial Deformities.* Vol. 3. Philadelphia, WB Saunders Company.
[20] Wilmot, J. J., Barber, H. D., Chou, D. G. & Vig, K. W. (1993). "Association between severity of dentofacial deformity and motivation for orthodontic orthognathic surgery treatment." *Angle Orthod*, 63, 283.
[21] Holtzman, L. S., Burns, E. R. & Kraut, R. A. (1992). "Preoperative laboratory assessment of hemostasis for orthognathic surgery." *Oral Surg Oral Med Oral Path*, 73, 403.
[22] Schultes, G., Gaggl, A. & Karcher, H. (1998). "Periodontal disease associated with interdental osteotomies after orthognathic surgery." *J Oral Maxillofac Surg*, 56, 414.
[23] Wolford, L. M. (1998). "Periodontal disease associated with interdental osteotomies after orthognathic surgery." *J Oral Maxillofac Surg*, 56, 417.
[24] Epker, B. N. & Fish, L. C. (1986). *Dentofacial deformities: Integrated Orthodontic & Surgical Correction.* Vol. 1, St. Louis, The C.V. Mosby Co.
[25] Arnett, G. W. & Bergman, R. T. (1993). "Facial keys to orthodontic diagnosis and treatment planning: Part II." *Am J Orthod Dentofac Orthop,* 103, 395-411.
[26] Farkas, L. G. (1981). *Anthropometry of head and face in medicine*. New York, Elsevier science Publishing Co.
[27] Talass, M. F. & Baker, R. C. (1987). "Soft tissue profile changes resulting from retraction of maxillary incisors." *Am J Orthod Dentofac Orthop*, 91, 385-394.
[28] Lo, F. D. & Hunter, W. S. (1982). "Changes in nasolabial angle related to maxillary incisor retraction." *Am J Orthod*, 82, 384-391.
[29] Holdaway, R. A. (1983). "A soft tissue cephalometric analysis and its use in orthodontic treatment planning: Part I." *Am J Orthod*, 84. 1-28.
[30] Oliver, B. M. (1982). "The influence of lip thickness and strain on upper lip response to incisor retraction." *Am J Orthod*, 82, 141-149.
[31] Peck, H. & Peck, S. (1970). "A concept of facial esthetics." *Angle Othod*, 40, 284-317.
[32] Burstone, C. J. (1967). "Lip posture and its significance in treatment planning." *Am J Orthod*, 53, 262-284.
[33] Clamon, L., Patton, D. & Rashid, R. (1990). "Standardized portrait photography for dental patients." *Am J Orthod*, 98, 197.
[34] Bell, W. H. & Scheindeman, G. B. (1981). "Correction of vertical maxillary deficiency: Stability and soft tissue changes." *J Oral Maxillofac Surg*, 39, 666-670.
[35] Burstone, C., James, R. B. & Legan, H. (1978). "Cepahlometrics for orthognathic surgery." *J Oral Surg*, 36, 269-277.
[36] Turvey, T. A. (1985). "Maxillary expansion: Technique based on surgical- orthodontic treatment objectives and anatomical considerations." *J Oral Maxillofac Surg*, 13, 51-58.
[37] Proffit, W. R., Phillips, C. & Turvey, T. A. (1987). "Stability following superior repositioning of maxilla by Le Fort I osteotomy." *Am J Orthod*, 92, 151-161.

[38] Finn, R. A., Throckmorton, G. S. & Bell, W. H. (1980). "Biomechanical considerations in the surgical correction of mandibular deficiency." *J Oral Surg*, 38, 257-264.

[39] Upton, P. M. (1997). "Evaluation of videoimaging prediction in combined maxillary and mandibular orthognathic surgery." *Am J Orthod*, 112, 656-665.

[40] Fish, L. C. & Epker, B. N. (1980). "Surgical orthodontic cephalometric prediction tracing." *J Clin Orthod*, 14, 36-52.

[41] Brewka, R. E. (1981). "Pantographic evaluation of cephalometric hinge axis." *Am J Orthod*, 79, 1-19.

[42] Sperry, T. P., Steinburg, M. J. & Gans, B. J. (1982). "Mandibular movement during autorotation as a result of maxillary impaction surgery." *Am J Orthod*, 81, 116-123.

[43] McCollum, T. G. (2001). "TOMAC: An orthognathic planning system: Part 2." *J Clin Orthod*, 35, 434-443.

[44] Sarver, D. & Johnston, M. W. (1988). "Videoimaging for planning and counseling in orthognathic surgery." *J Oral Maxillofac Surg*, 46, 939-945.

[45] Sarver, D. (1997). *Esthetics in Orthodontics and Orthognathic Surgery.* St. Louis, Mosby - Year Book.

[46] Sarver, D. (1996). "Videocephalometrics diagnosis: A new concept in treatment planning?" *Am J Orthod*, 110, 128-136.

[47] Hohl, T., Wolford, L. M., Epker, B. N. & Fonseca, R. J. (1978). "Craniofacial osteotomies – A photocephalometric technique for prediction and evaluation of tissue change." *Angle Orthod*, 48, 114-125.

[48] Phillips, C., Hill, B. & Cannac, C. (1995). "The influence of videoimaging on patient's perceptions and expectations." *Angle Orthod*, 107, 177-185.

[49] Sarver, D. & Johnston, M. W. (1993). "Orthognathic surgery and esthetics: planning treatment to achieve functional and esthetic goals." *Br J Orthod*, 20: 93-100.

[50] Sinclair, P. M., Kilpelainen, P. & Phillips, C. (1995). "The accuracy of videoimaging in orthognathic surgery." *Am J Orthod*, 107, 177-185.

[51] Jacobs, J. D. & Sinclair, P. M. (1984). "Principles of orthodontic mechanics in orthognathic surgery cases." *Am J Orthod*, 184, 399-407.

[52] Lines, P. A. & Steinhauser, E W. (1974). "Diagnosis and treatment planning in surgical orthodontic therapy." *Am J Orthod*, 66, 378-397.

AUTHORS' CONTACT INFORMATION

Dr. Devinder Preet Singh, B.D.S, M.D.S (Orthodontics)
Senior Lecturer
Department Of Orthodontics & Dentofacial Orthopedics
Dr. Harvansh Singh Judge Institute of Dental Sciences
Sector 25, South Campus, Panjab University, Chandigarh
E-mail: ahluwalia147@gmail.com

Dr. Shefali Arora, B.D.S, M.D.S (Oral Surgery)
Senior Lecturer
Department of Oral & Maxillofacial Surgery
Swami Devi Dyal Dental College & Hospital
Barwala, Panchkula, Haryana
E-mail: shefalina@rediffmail.com

INDEX

A

B

C

D

E

F

G

H

I

J

L

M

N

O

P

Q

R

S

T

V

W